P9-DDU-889

Date Due

RC   Mount, James L.
622   The food and health
M68   of Western man /
       James Lambert Mount.

Stockton State College
Library
Pomona, N. J. 08240

The Food and Health of Western Man

The Food and Health of Western Man

James Lambert Mount, B.A., M.B., M.R.C.P.

A HALSTED PRESS BOOK

JOHN WILEY & SONS
New York

Published in the U.S.A.
by Halsted Press, a Division
of John Wiley & Sons, Inc.,
New York

© 1975 James Lambert Mount

Library of Congress Cataloging in Publication Data

Mount, James Lambert
   The food and health of Western man

   "A Halsted Press book"
   1. Deficiency diseases. 2. Nutrition
I. Title. [DNLM: 1. Nutrition. 2. Health. QU145 M926f]
RC620.5.M68   616.3'9   75-11989
ISBN 0-470-61957-0

Printed in Great Britain

STOCKTON STATE COLLEGE LIBRARY
POMONA, NEW JERSEY 08240

To my Mother and my Father

The greatest single factor in the
acquisition and maintenance of
good health is perfectly
constituted food.

Sir Robert McCarrison

Contents

Preface

This book is written from a deep concern felt by the author concerning the health of western civilised man. Very important changes are occurring in the way we live and way we eat and these are affecting the overall pattern of disease. Certain chronic diseases are increasing in prevalence remarkably and this can be shown largely to be due to the food we eat and the increase in consumption of certain foodstuffs, over the past seventy years particularly.

Food is richer, softer and sweeter than ever before. Food is richer because we eat more fat, softer because it is processed to a high degree and has lost its natural fibre (together with other factors), and food is sweeter from our greatly increased consumption of sugar. The transition of a foodstuff from a raw unprocessed state to a processed state involves loss of nutrients including trace elements, minerals and vitamins. All these factors together add up to a very significant change in quality of food eaten today and the total nutriture afforded by such food.

Comparing a diet based on refined sugar, refined flour, over-consumption of fried foods, processed vegetables, canned fruits and processed dehydrated potatoes to a diet based upon, for instance, wholegrain cereals, fresh milk, fresh fruit, and raw vegetables, one does not need a computer to sense the difference. Meat, scarce as it is, becomes less of a necessity if the diet is wholesome and well balanced. This is now becoming acknowledged by the most diehard of nutritionists. However, the evidence is that the diet is *not* well balanced at this time, and the imbalance derives from certain areas of nutrition.

The snack food and confectionery trades have multiplied

enormously of recent years. The excess intake of sugar and fat based upon poor quality food material from these sources affects young people especially. Crisps, lollipops, sweets, biscuits and refined flour products are eaten in abundance by children. The obvious damage to health resulting from this is seen in the appalling state of children's teeth today. This can only reflect a poor state of nutrition generally in the child. Much evidence concerning this is presented later in the book. This is but one example of the influence that food technology has had upon the state of health of the people. Food technology obviously in itself is not bad; it is the way, rather, that the populace succumb to its blandishments. Food technology has its place, and a very important place, in the handling and redistribution of food, but abuse of this branch of science could lead to nutritional disaster. In this book a change to more wholesome food is very seriously advocated if chronic ill health is not to become a permanent deficiency of westernised nations.

Arguments against such conclusions usually state that (1) there is no evidence, and (2) the change-over would be too expensive for the population to bear. In answer to the first point this book has been written. In answer to the second, it can be said that if the motivation is there the way can be found. What is more precious to a household, their purchase of a colour T.V. set or the purchase of their health? A headline appeared in the *Daily Mail* of February 7th, 1973 stating 'Mrs. 1973 puts holiday and new car before food'. The article reported that the average expenditure on food had dropped from 29.5% to 20% in ten years. The longer holiday, the colour T.V., the car, the Bingo hall and the betting shop are more exciting ways of spending money than buying food, and food purchase has as a consequence dropped. If Mrs. 1973 put her mind to it she could feed herself and her family more healthily and not a great deal more expensively *if* the education and the motivation were there. Technology should serve a public, not bind it or dominate it. The time has come when existing trends must be reversed, or, if not reversed, at least adjusted to, or man will not survive to obtain a healthy state.

In all that has been said, it is fully realised by the author that food is not the only factor which causes disease. The psychology of man, his mental health, his happiness and his contentment with his work are probably more potent factors than any in the promotion of health. It has not been the purpose of this book to weigh these or even contrast these factors. They are there and their presence is acknowledged. The axiom that 'man does not live by bread alone' is as true here as of any other area of life. Man's total state of well-being depends upon man's total environment. Man's psychological state is one of the most important factors affecting his health. His nutrition is another. It is the wish of the author that this book might contribute in a small way to the greater understanding of man's health and the factors that affect it.

One

Food yesterday and today

Food habits are changing, fast. For society itself is changing and social structures with it. Technology is developing and the deep ingrained social habits of centuries are being influenced, modified and remoulded. New foods are appearing, new ways of preparing and processing food are being introduced. Indeed food can now be stored, transported, altered, processed, rejuvenated, texturised or flavoured whereas before it could only be eaten! The way too we eat food has radically altered over the last seventy years. Meals are taken differently and in new environments. Time taken in the preparing and eating of food is less. Convenience is the factor primarily sought, and that which is paid for. All this must affect the state of man's health for man's nutrition is intimately related to his health.

Sir Jack Drummond[7] in his interesting and well-known book, *The Englishman's Food*, traces the origin of our eating over many centuries. As much a social commentary, as a nutritional one, the book is fascinating for the insight it gives into the lives of our ancestors, their poverty, their wealth and their eating. The book is the primary reference for material presented in the first section of this chapter, and should be referred to for a more complete commentary upon the history of eating and nutrition of our own land.

Poverty of nutrition is not new

The first point that is made by Sir Jack Drummond in his book is that poverty of nutrition has been prevalent in this island over many centuries and was severe as recently as 70 years ago. The years 1880—1910 saw more disease from malnutrition in this country than perhaps at any other time. Indeed the poor have always eaten badly and the poor have always been with us.

The contrast between 70 years ago and the present day has been summarised as a shift merely from 'diseases of undernutrition' to 'diseases of overnutrition'. Whereas before, people suffered on poor quality bread and cheese, nowadays they suffer on poor quality bread, sugar and processed foods! A century ago it could be said the lower social classes suffered from an undersupply of poor quality foods. Nowadays they suffer from oversupply of similarly poor quality foods. This is obviously an oversimplification but it makes a point which will be more thoroughly examined throughout this book.

Bread, beef, beer and cheese

The second theme that sounds through Drummond's book shows that four foods were the foundation of the Englishman's diet, bread, beef, beer and cheese. It is interesting to reflect that these same four foods are those that appear most frequently in the English pub today, though in a considerably watered-down version! The bread, before the year 1870, was made from coarse stone-ground flour and though often whitened in the towns with such adulterates as alum or potato flour it mostly contained its full quota of nutrients. This was perhaps fortunate as bread often comprised 70%, of total calorie intake for some of the very poor who could not afford better. Beer was home brewed and strong. A small beer of two hundred years ago has been estimated to have contained 150 - 200 calories per pint, and a moderate supply of calcium, riboflavin, nicotinic acid and B vitamins with it. Children also drank beer.

Brief historical survey

17th century

Time of Expansion. Impetus to Agriculture.

Farming consisting of corn-growing, some dairy cattle.

Art of gardening flourishing.

Vegetables and Fruit grown for the rich.

Tea, coffee and chocolate introduced in late 17th century.

Diet of the rich:

Breakfast of cold meats, fish (salted herrings), cheese and ale.

Dinner midday of 'hot shoulder of mutton', 'cold chine of roast beef', or a 'good dish of roasted chicken', served with ale and cheese.

Vegetables were being introduced with servings.

Diet of the poor:

Bread, beef, beer and cheese, or if times were hard:

Bread and coarse vegetable broth.

18*th century*

1st half—prosperous.

2nd half—poverty from poor harvests and trading difficulties.

Increase in agricultural efficiency brought increase in milk, butter, vegetables and bread.

Vegetables were brought to the towns.

Northerners were experimenting with potatoes.

Change and disruption beginning in village life.

Much wine and beer drunk.

'Puddings' were becoming popular.

A French commentator of the time writes:

'Blessed be he that invented Pudding for it is a Manna that hits the Palates of all sorts of People!!'

Monsieur Misson's Memoirs (1719)

Sugar became available.

19*th century*

Industrialisation speeding up.

Over-crowding in towns, poor hygiene.

War. Financial and trade disturbances.

Poor harvests. Hunger rioting 1815-1819.

Engels[8] describes the factory children as 'hollow-eyed ghosts' riddled with scrofula and rickets.

Later half:

Agricultural and Industrial Expansion.

Birth of the Food Industry.

Sugar consumption rockets.

Tea consumption rockets.

Main foods: potatoes, meat, bread.

Chief food of townspeople: bread.

An analysis of the diet of 19 working class families in 1841 reveals the quality of food consumed:

3

Food	Amount consumed per head per week	Percentage contribution to			Comment
		Calories	Protein	Iron	
Flour					$\frac{1}{3}$ of food
(Bread)	5 lb	50	40	40	expenditure
Potatoes	5 lb	20	20		Some vitamin C available
Meat	1 lb		25	20	$\frac{1}{6}$ of food expenditure
Sugar	7 oz				

Source: J. C. McKenzie[13]

This great reliance on bread is shown by the fact that in 1892 children in Bethnal Green were nourished almost entirely upon bread, 83% of them having no other solid food in 17 out of 21 meals of the week. This threw a heavy onus of responsibility on the nutrients in bread to preserve health. This is discussed in more detail in the chapter on bread but it is in context here to say a little about the effect that was wrought by the introduction of the roller mills in the 1870s upon bread and nutrition.

Bread
Iron roller mills for grinding flour had been patented by Wilkinson as long ago as 1753 though it was not till the introduction of porcelain in 1870 that such machines were found to be serviceable. In 1877 encouraged by what they had seen in Budapest and Vienna a group of Englishmen led by Lord Radford of Liverpool set up roller mills in this country. They proliferated so fast that within a very few years the mills had almost superseded the age old process of stone grinding flour. Reasons for this rapid expansion were not hard to find. The roller milling was quick, economical and efficient. Degree of milling could be nicely controlled to produce as white a flour as was demanded by the public and the public liked white flour. It is a delusion to believe that white bread was forced upon an unwilling public. Ever since Roman times

4

white flour carried a premium value. Symbol of wealth and purity, it was always the richest who could afford it while the poor ate the darker bread. Townsmen particularly had always had a strong preference for white bread.

However a subtle and very important difference was introduced with roller milling. Previously the inefficiency of refining white flour through muslin and linen fabrics had retained a fair amount of wheat germ in the flour—hence the yellow creamy colour of such flour. The efficiency of the roller mills could separate out the wheat germ completely and produce a whiter flour, *though a flour devoid of germ.* The germ is that part of the wheat seed that surrounds the plumule (the new wheat shoot) and the radicle (the new root). It is therefore that part of the wheat seed that contains most of the nutrients for plant development in a readily available form. These nutrients include most of the B vitamins, vitamin E and also a better quality protein than is found in the starchy endosperm. But the germ also contained fats, and essential fatty acids and here lay the rub. Fats meant poor keeping quality and the development of rancid flour if flour was kept too long. The millers did not want the germ for this reason and were only too happy to sacrifice it in the interests of a whiter flour that also stored better. Desire for white bread had thus laid its own nutritional trap.

Drummond estimates that the milling depleted the diet of the poor of .7 mg B_1 (daily requirement 1.2 mg) 4 mg nicotinic acid (daily requirement 12 mg) 4 mg iron (daily requirement 12 mg) certain essential fats, minerals (from the husk) and good quality protein. A largish sacrifice had been paid. No doubt partly due to this fact, though how much it is very hard to say, and partly due to factors of overcrowding, poor hygiene and sanitation, the end of the 19th century saw a marked decline in the health and physique of townspeople. The glories of the empire abroad were a contrast to the inglorious state of our health at home! An average of 40% of all recruits (60% in some locations) called up for the South African war at the end of the 19th century were rejected on grounds of deformities, heart affections, poor sight, hearing and rotten teeth[19]. The matter was reported to Whitehall and a full government enquiry was held which confirmed the poor state of health of such people[17].

Preparation for the 20*th century*
It can be said truly that the country had paid a hard price for industrialisation. Such diseases as tuberculosis, dysentery, typhoid and diphtheria were rife in the cities and deficiency diseases common. An estimate was made that a third of poor children at the time were suffering from rickets. Dental health deteriorated. Vitamin A and C deficiencies were common. The thirty years following 1880 in fact saw perhaps some of the worst malnutrition this country has ever known.

Against this must be set in contrast the general improvement in diet of the upper classes and the maintenance of fair health amongst the countryfolk. The rich seemed to be eating richer, the poor were eating poorer, while the countryfolk maintained two important safeguards to their health, their country-milled flour and their own vegetables. The staple diet of the Englishman was still bread, meat, butter and cheese but to this were now added tea, sugar, and some vegetables. These latter were now accepted as a reasonable accompaniment to a meat dish though foreigners would express distress if not horror at the way we English cooked them:

> The English system of cooking it would be impertinent of me to describe; but still when I think of that huge round of par-boiled ox flesh, with sodden dumplings floating in a saline, greasy mixture, surrounded by carrots looking red with disgust, and turnips pale with dismay, I cannot help a sort of inward shudder, and the making of comparisons unfavourable to English gastronomy.[18]

The picture is familiar!

Throughout the 19th century milk production increased, and in the North particularly the growing of potatoes and oats contributed significantly to the diet. The Scottish labourer of the time was much better fed than his English counterpart. Food was part of his wage and this food largely consisted of oats (porridge), milk and vegetables—a good diet. His strong physique was commented upon at the time and contrasted to the puny Englishman! It is interesting to reflect on how many of our empire pioneers were Scottish in origin, and brought up on the oats and milk of their land.

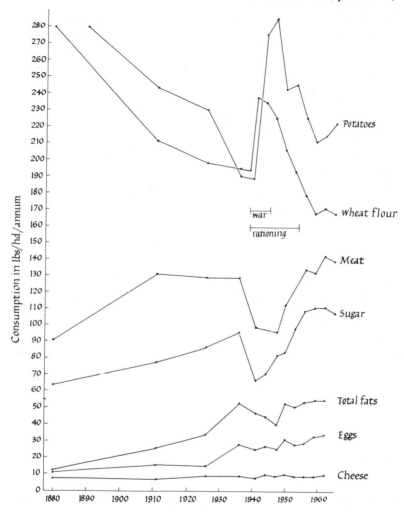

1.1. Consumption of principal foodstuffs in U.K. 1880-1965 (from Greaves J.P. and Hollingsworth D. F., *World Review Nutrition and Dietetics*, 1966, 6 : 34)

From 1910 social and welfare improvements stimulated an improvement in health. Hygiene and nutrition followed suit. In the 1920s many of the vitamins were outlined and discovered and nutritional science was born. The nutritional story now entered a new phase.

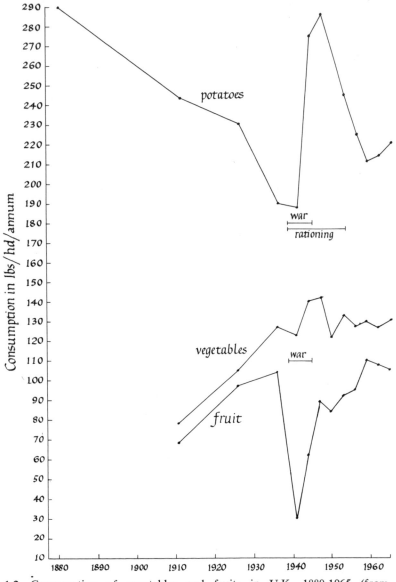

1.2 Consumption of vegetables and fruits in U.K. 1880-1965 (from Greaves J.P. and Hollingsworth D. F., *World Review Nutrition and Dietetics,* 1966, 6:34)

The last 70 *years.* (See Figs. 1.1 and 1.2)

The diet for the average Briton within the last 70 years has become richer, sweeter, more varied, and more refined.

Protein consumption has increased over a 'wide front'.

Milk, meat, eggs have increased in their consumption.

Potato and bread have decreased (monotonous bulky food).

Fibre has been refined out of the diet.

Sugar has increased greatly, especially in lower classes, replacing bread and potato.

Butter and Fat consumption have increased.

Vegetables and Fruit have increased.

Refined foods, conserved and packeted foods have greatly increased.

Differences in food consumption are now far less between classes.

Analysis of some of these trends in further details now follows.

Sugar and carbohydrates

In 1226 Henry III asked the Mayor of Winchester to procure for him 3 lb of Alexandria sugar 'if so much could be got'. At a later date it is known that in 1319 a shipment of sugar was received in London, in exchange for wool. In the following centuries as trade gradually increased and prices fell, consumption slowly rose and was standing at 4 lb/person/year at the beginning of the 18th century. In 1845 consumption was 20 lb/person/year and a meteoric rise brought this figure up to 93 lb/person in 1901 (with removal of tax duties). The current figure now stands at 126 lb/person/year. The United Kingdom is at present exceeded in sugar consumption by only four countries: Greenland, Gibraltar, Iceland and Hawaii!

Reasons for this rise in sugar consumption are probably various. Apart from the obvious reason that sugar is sweet and attractive (and experimental animals also grow fat on it by choice) sugar is a useful preservative for jams, fruits and vegetables. It is also widely used in soups and of course pastries, to increase palatability. However apart from its various metabolic reactions which are being detailed in present day science, sugar is the great deceiver.[20] It displaces from the diet not only the complex carbohydrates, potato and bread, but also other more worthwhile foods such as meat, vegetables and fruit. For sugar satiates the appetite and deceives the palate. The supply of certain vitamins and

9

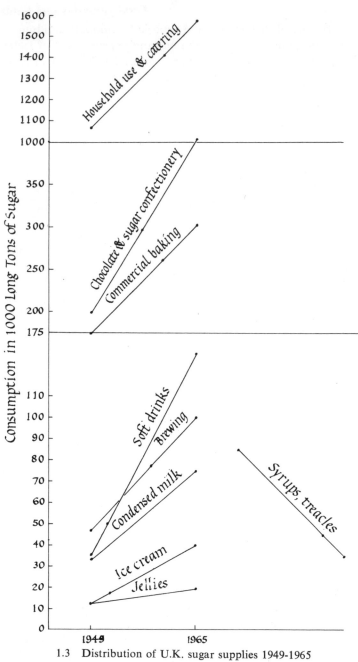

1.3   Distribution of U.K. sugar supplies 1949-1965

minerals is thus placed at risk and especially amongst children.

It is interesting to see how the use and consumption of sugar is divided and in what manufacture it is used (Fig. 1.3.) Confectionery, ice cream, soft drinks, household use of sugar have all

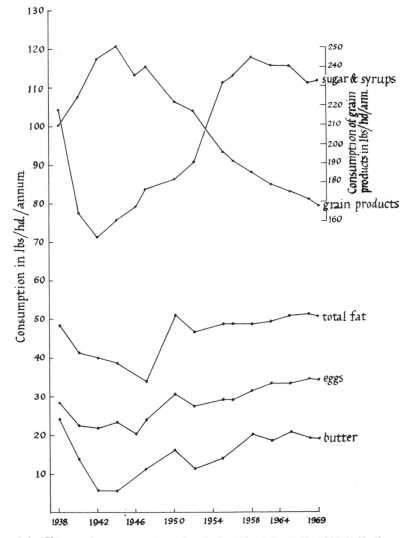

1.4 Changes in consumption of principal food in U.K. 1938-1969 (from *Household Food Consumption and Expenditure*, Ministry of Agric. Fish Food 1969)

11

increased. Jams and syrups have declined. Sugar now contributes *twice* as big a proportion by weight to total carbohydrates as in 1944, *thirty* years ago.

The universal change in consumption from complex carbohydrates of bread and potato to the simple carbohydrates of sugar is shown for this country (Fig. 1.4) and for America (Fig. 1.5). In both countries bread and potatoes provided about 44% of calorie intake in 1910 and just half that figure in 1964. Bread is

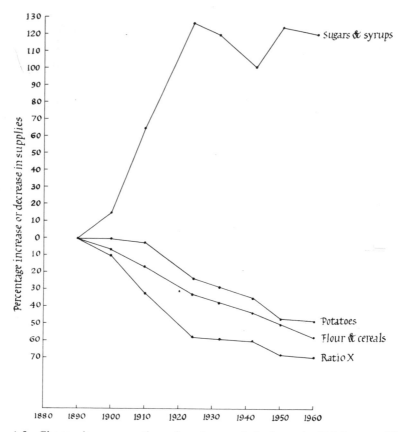

1.5 Change in consumption of various carbohydrates in U.S.A. over 80 years (from **Antar M. A., Ohlson M. A., Hodges R. E.,** *Amer. J. Clin.*

Nutr., 1964, 14:169 x: Ratio x = $\dfrac{\text{Complex carbohydrate}}{\text{Simple carbohydrate}}$

declining in popularity. No doubt much of this decline as has been said is due to the increased richness as also the variability of our diet. There are so many more attractive foods available to eat. Part of the decline however may be due to the decrease in palatability of modern bread, though this is hard to prove.

Oatmeal, like bread, is another complex carbohydrate on the decline. The traditional Scottish porridge breakfast is giving way to the breakfast cereal. Breakfast cereals have trebled in consumption over ten years, and are another example of an outlet for sugar. 4,300 tons of sugar were used in their manufacture in 1949 and several thousand tons more in the eating of them. The amount may have doubled since that year. Porridge and milk has been stated to be one of the most nutritious of common food combinations. Breakfast cereals are nutritionally a very poor substitute for these two foods.

Different metabolic reactions within the body follow the consumption of starch, a complex carbohydrate, as opposed to sucrose, a disaccharide and simple carbohydrate. These will be discussed later in the book. It is sufficient at the moment to state that this particular change in the constitution of our diet may be the *most important* that has taken place in 100 years.

The potato's place in modern nutrition is also shrinking. Consumption is falling though it shows signs of having found its level. The potato still contributes substantially to the overall nutrition of the nation. 37% of our vitamin C intake, 14% of our vitamin B1, 13% of our nicotinic acid, 9% of our carbohydrates, 9% of our iron and 5% of our protein is contributed by the potato. More still of our minerals and vitamins would be supplied by this vegetable if not eaten so frequently as chips or crisps. 50% of the vitamin C content of the potato is lost in eating it as a chip and 90% as crisps. Minerals and a certain amount of protein are lost on peeling, for as with the wheat seed, large quantities of these nutrients reside within the skin layer. A large segment of the population rely on the potato nevertheless to supply up to 75% of their daily vitamin C requirement.

Refining of carbohydrates

By refining processes, bread, rice and potatoes are made whiter, softer and smoother. The most important nutritional ingredient lost to the human body through such a process is fibre. A pro-

13

portion of fibre has been lost overall from the diet over the past 70 years in comparison to rises in consumption of fats and sugar. Certain chronic diseases of the alimentary tract, diverticulosis and colonic cancer for instance can be shown to occur as a result and conditions such as haemorrhoids, varicose veins and obesity are encouraged. Some authorities consider the loss of this nutrient more disastrous than any other change in our nutrition of late years (see Chapter 10).

Meat and protein
The protein value of the diet has increased in 70 years and more meat has been eaten. Over the last 10 years beef consumption has dropped and poultry meat from broilers increased threefold. A further increase is likely. Fish has decreased in popularity despite increase in purchase of prepared frozen fish (which accounts for 20% of all fish landings at the present moment). Eggs have increased in consumption and probably account for some of the drop in beef sales. Eggs now contribute significantly within the population to vitamin A sources (8%), riboflavin (7%), iron (7%), calcium and protein. Meat itself provides half our nicotinic acid and a third of our fat and iron.

Oils and fats
Total fat consumption increased considerably in the first part of this century and between 1910 and 1936 the population doubled its consumption of fat. Consumption of margarine increased alongside butter up till 1952 but since that year has given way to butter. Concerning the controversy as to which fats are beneficial to health, animal or vegetable it is pertinent to note that 82% of our fat is animal, and 18% vegetable. Over the past 50 years consumption of fat has increased by 100% While total fat intake over this period has doubled, essential fatty acid intake has only risen from 10 g to 14 g per day, a small rise by proportion. The difference in quality of fats is further explained in the chapter on heart disease. Essential fatty acids are 'unsaturated' and of greater physiological use to the body. They are contained in more abundance in vegetable fats and contribute to the nutritional superiority of vegetable over animal fats. Milk, meat, eggs and butter provide most of our animal fat in the diet.

14

Rise in consumption of sucrose has in some countries paralleled rise in consumption of fat. As both foodstuffs are incriminated in heart disease (and obesity and diabetes) it is difficult to discriminate, epidemiologically, between the two. Foods such as ice cream contain both products and ice cream for instance doubled its national consumption between 1956 and 1965.

Geographical and social differences
Variations in food consumption exist between different areas of the country. One of the most interesting of these variations is that found between Scotland and Southern England (as also Scotland and Wales). Scotland is a country addicted to high teas and puddings. Southern England, on the other hand, consumes more fruit and vegetable. Whether the Scottish diet is a legacy from the days when battles were fought on porridge is hard to say, but far less fruit and vegetable is consumed in North England and Scotland than Southern England! The National Food Survey[10] shows these differences and comments upon them. Higher than the national average, were the consumption levels of cakes, biscuits, margarine, suet, dripping, preserves and ready-made bread, in Scotland. Lower than anywhere else were consumption levels of vegetables and fruit. Consumption of fresh fruit was 24% below the national average and fresh vegetables 60% below this average. The Ministry report comments upon the very low intakes of vitamin C in Scotland. Vegetable intake being small, Scotsmen also suffered low intakes of vitamin A.

Characteristics of the Scottish diet are also repeated in the North of England where high consumption of cakes and biscuits and low consumption of fresh fruits and green vegetables lead to lower essential vitamin intakes than average. In Chapter 8 which deals with Britain's health it will be seen that Scotland has the shortest life expectancy in Europe.

Class distinctions still exist as regards food consumption and in this direction the accusation is often made that the labouring class eat badly and exist on fish and chips and cups of tea. Some years ago E. M. Bramwell[2] carried out a survey of the diet habits of London busmen to assess the truth of the matter. They did not eat a great deal of fish and chips but their food habits were revealing. There was a general liking found for simple plain food, and regular habits of eating. A low consumption of fruit and

15

vegetables was also noted. The eating routine was as follows:

Breakfast:	50% had tea, bread, butter
	50% had either cereals or cooked breakfast
Midday meal:	Meat, egg or fish with vegetables (Meat pies were more common than fish)
	Pudding taken regularly was fruit tart or fruit and custard
Snacks a.m., p.m.:	Tea, biscuits, sometimes fruit cake
At night:	Snack (Breakfast cereals, or bacon and egg or bread)
	Tea.

Calories provided by the Busman's diet

Bread and butter	25%
Protein foods	20%
Milk, sugar	20%
Biscuits, cakes	10%
Potatoes	5%
Puddings	4%
Veg., fruits	3%

Consumption of tea averaged 45 cups a week (7 a day) with a minimum of 11 and a maximum of 95 cups a week! A low consumption of fruit and vegetables was noted but unfortunately no assessment accompanies the survey, of actual vitamin C intake, which therefore must remain conjectural. The diet shows a heavy reliance upon bread, butter, milk, meat, eggs and sugar. However at least these men were eating cooked food and food cooked reasonably fresh for there are indications that cooked food will soon be replaced by precooked and processed meals sold from the vending machine.

In America such is occurring. E. J. Lease et al.[11] in a study of the midday meal of industrial workers in the U.S.A. found that the canteen lunch was giving way to the snack supplied by such a vending machine. Full meals were eaten less and such foods as meat dishes, vegetables and salads were omitted as a result. Snacks tend to consist of 'filler foods' and on the whole constitute second-class foods rather than first-class and as a result overall standards of nutrition suffer.

Emphasis is given to further change in eating habits in the United States by a recent report issued by the U.S. Department of Agriculture. The secretary of this organisation, Orville Freeman[14] has been quoted as stating that in America 20% of families are now inadequately feeding themselves. This figure was 15% ten years ago and Freeman states that there has been a deterioration in nutritional standards in ten years. Over ten years there has been an increase in consumption of *sweet rolls, cakes, soft drinks and meat*. There has been a decrease in the amount of milk, fruit and vegetables eaten. A finding reported in this statement that caused some interest was the estimate that 9% of upper income families fell below required nutritional standards and 30% in the lower income bracket. Wealth does not necessarily lead to health. Nutritional standards are for the most part arbitrarily fixed and allow margins of safety so too much attention cannot therefore be paid to individual assessment ratings but overall trends do not lie and it is alarming that 5% of the American population are worse fed now than ten years ago.

Magnus Pyke in a recent article in the *New Scientist*[16] is optimistic over future nutritional standards to be achieved by populations consuming new types of processed foods. At the moment there are few grounds for optimism. Advances in America generally foreshadow advances in the rest of the civilised world and the reports of nutritional betterment, freedom from disease and greater health in this first nation of the world are *not* evident. They should be. Some rethinking might soon be necessary if 2000 A.D. is to be our Utopia.

Convenience foods and social habits

The term convenience foods as used by the National Food Survey includes all bottled, canned, packeted and processed foods on the market. Fig. 1.6 shows the rise in consumption of these foods that has taken place in ten years. The proportion of the national food expenditure given to the purchase of such foods was 17% in 1956, and 20% in 1965; not in fact a great rise and less than in America. However the figures are not complete for the National Food Survey only covers food eaten at home and more meals and snacks are being eaten away from home than previously. The proportion of expenditure given to them is also increasing.

Fig. 1.6 shows the rapid rise in consumption of quick frozen

17

The food and health of western man

fish, quick frozen peas and beans and canned soups that has taken place in ten years. The fish, and peas (and crisps) have quadrupled, and canned soups trebled. Dehydrated soups have almost trebled. The rise in consumption of fruit juices and canned fruits has detracted from the sale of fresh fruit. Quick frozen peas and beans have similarly displaced fresh vegetables. In a survey conducted by

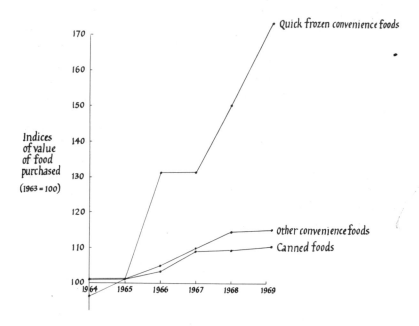

1.6 Indices of value of convenience foods purchased for household consumption 1964-1969 (from *Household Food Consumption and Expenditure: 1969*, H.M.S.O. 1971)

the Food Education Society canned fruit proved the most popular dessert[4], being more popular than fresh fruit.

The National Food Survey reports an increase in cakes and pastries bought for the home, ice creams and prepared puddings. Snack foods bought outside the home are not included in the survey but biscuit production has doubled in the ten years and one independent survey estimated that three out of every five people eat five or more biscuits a day[5].

Teenagers consume many of these foods and M. Abrams[1] in an

18

independent survey found that 12% of a teenager's income was spent on snacks, sweets and soft drinks. Teenagers as a group accounted for 15% of all consumer spending on sweets and 20% of all spending on soft drinks. Teenagers, as will be shown later in the book, are a group prone to bad eating habits and the consumption of snacks.

Evidence of ignorance also exists amongst housewives. The results of one survey reported in the bulletin of the Food Education Society[3] showed that only one woman in five knows why vitamins are essential to the diet. Those over 35 in age were the most knowledgeable, the younger housewife the most ignorant. Social changes have taken place fast in the last 15 years and food habits have changed almost as quickly.

40-50% of housewives go out to work and rely on quick evening purchases in the supermarket and grocery store on their way home. Convenience sells a food best, rapidity and ease of preparation being qualities that rate the highest. Taste comes next and nutritional value is of low importance or not rateable due to ignorance! Time spent preparing food and time spent in the kitchen is time wasted in the estimation of many modern-day housewives. One housewife put it well enough in a report carried by a local paper recently[12]:

> My husband insists that we buy fresh vegetables, but by the time I have fiddled about preparing it and throwing quite a lot away, it would have been just as good to have opened a packet of peas.

This particular housewife said that if she was given the choice she would always use frozen food and this seems to be the trend amongst younger housewives. In the same article in this paper another young housewife stated that because she was at work all day she used frozen and tinned food during the week. But when the weekend came, she and her husband desired a more elaborate meal and used fresh fruit and vegetables with a traditional Sunday joint. A prominent processing company, Birds Eye, now claim one third of the total national acreage of peas and green beans!

The frozen food trade will no doubt expand a great deal in years to come. Already in America the output of such foods has passed 10,000 million lb (in 1939 total output was but 325 million lb). Vegetables and poultry provide a quarter of this amount, potatoes 8%, peas 16%. Fruit juices and concentrates are the next largest item closely followed by the prepared foods (fruit pies and meat pies). It is in this last item, concerning precooked foods, that the future expansion of the industry is considered to lie[9].

On the whole nutritional quality, the vitamin and mineral content of frozen food, is good, better certainly than much canned food or food that has been dehydrated. However with any processing treatment there is danger that unobserved nutrients are lost. *When more and more of our food is subjected to some form of precooking, processing or preserving treatment there is the likelihood that more and more essential nutrients such as vitamins, minerals and certain trace factors will be whittled away to cause some form of deficiency.* This must always be a potential danger if not yet actually realised. The destruction of certain taste factors also leads to change in flavour. One of the most subtle dangers that derives from refined foods is the deception of the palate by sweetening agents and flavours which encourage overconsumption of poor quality foods.

Food chemistry will expand and nutritional science will evolve. There is always the hope that the latter science will keep an eye on the former, eradicate the disadvantages that follow from the former and in its turn lend advice that will confer nutritional advantages upon future reforms. One would hope for this anyway, because the changes that J. G. Davis[6] forecasts for the next century are dramatic. They could be damaging. Looking ahead to 2000 A.D., Davis, past Chairman of the Society of Chemical Industry Food Group, makes some of the following predictions for our civilisation:

(1) Economic synthesis of amino acids, proteins.
(2) Economic synthesis of sugars, fats, carbohydrates.
(3) Economic synthesis of all known vitamins and flavours.
(4) Efficient extraction of protein from leaves and waste vegetable matter and the making of protein by micro-organisms.
(5) All foods to be consumed from packages (plastic and long keeping).
(6) Prepared meals to be provided by vending machines.
(7) The diet to be a blend of 'natural' derivatives (e.g. leaf protein) and 'artificial' (e.g. synthesised fat).
     We shall see!

20

Food yesterday and today

An attempt has been made in this chapter to show the dramatic changes occurring within the diet of our time. It has been said that we have moved from one phase of malnutrition into another, from undernutrition to overnutrition, and all within the space of seventy years. Dramatic have been the changes in quality of food and these are assessed in detail in this book. Our diet is too rich, too sweet and too soft and is disease-contributing.

REFERENCES TO CHAPTER 1

1 Abrams M., *The Teenage Consumer,* London Press Exchange Ltd., London 1959.
2 Bramwell E. M., *Proc. Nutr. Soc. (Lond.)* 1961, 20: 30.
3 *Bulletin of the Food Education Society,* June 1966. F.E.S., 190 Piccadilly, W.1.
4 ——May 1968. F.E.S., 190 Piccadilly, W.1.
5 ——July 1967. F.E.S., 190 Piccadilly, W.1.
6 Davis J. G., *J. Roy. Soc. Arts* 1966, 114: 64.
7 Drummond J., Wilbraham A., *The Englishman's Food,* Cape, London. 1957.
8 Engels F., *The Condition of the Working Class in England in* 1844. First English Edition 1892, cited by Drummond p.307.
9 Franklin A. F., *Quick Frozen Foods* 1963, 26: 41.
10 Household Food Consumption and Expenditure for 1965, *Annual report of the National Food Survey Committee* H.M.S.O., London. 1967.
11 Lease E. J., Anderson H. S., Malphus R. K., Lease J. G., *J. Amer. Diet Ass.* 1963, 43: 34.
12 *Loughton Express* Aug. 16, 1968.
13 McKenzie J. C., *Proc. Nutr. Soc.* (Lond.) 1966, 25. No. 1 XIV.
14 *Medical News,* Mar. 15, 1968.
15 Natural Food and Farming, *Journal of the Natural Food Associates,* July 1968. Atlanta, Texas.
16 Pyke M., *New Scientist* 1969, 42: 468, May 29th.
17 Report of the Inter-Departmental Committee on Physical Deterioration 1904, cited by Drummond p.404.
18 *The Memoirs of a Stomach,* edited by Minister of the Interior, 4th ed., 1853, cited by Drummond p.334.
19 Welt Smyth A., *Physical Deterioration, its cause and cure.* 1907, cited by Drummond p.404.
20 Yudkin J., *The Lancet* 1963, 1: 1335.

Two

Food processing
and irradiation

Food must be processed to be distributed. This goes without saying. Large urban conurbations separate country from town and means have to be found to store, process, packet and transport the food to the city dweller. Fresh food is a luxury and often an impossibility under such circumstances.

Modern science has conveniently come to the aid of the food distributor and today's supermarket presents as much a triumph of food engineering and processing as can anywhere be found. However the great and obvious danger is that the processing gimmick goes to the food manufacturer's head and all for the sake of commercial gain. There is no doubt that fish fingers are more popular than fresh fish. That does not mean that they are more nutritious. There comes a stage when the total quantity of nutrients, refined, processed, bleached and irradiated out of our food begins to take its toll upon the human constitution. The manufacturer is not *basically* concerned with this problem. He is primarily geared to sell his product and make a profit. Providing the product has some nutrients retained and a sufficient taste to ensure commercial success, which taste can always be modified by a chemical additive, he is clear. *But any processing procedure must by its nature deprive the food of some of its nutrient.* Many of them such as irradiation alter the food to a high degree, other procedures to a lesser degree. There are many ingredients in food that are still undetected, unanalysed and unplaced. What exactly differentiates fresh food from stale food or fresh food from processed foods? Essential oils? Vitamins? Essential fatty acids? How important are the trace factors in food? What is a healthy food? All these questions are difficult to answer. Nutrition in many ways is an infant science and has many areas of development yet to explore.

Urban development and city life make the consumption of fresh fruit and vegetables, locally grown, less possible. Technology provides more refined techniques every day for processing food but these extravagances of processing must be curbed. Mistakes are inevitably made. Chemicals are used which should not be used and the balance of the diet is significantly altered. There is often no restraint till too late. Nutritional science can just not keep pace with processing and marketing procedures. There are 2,000 additives allowed or used in food processing at the present moment. Only a few of these have been *thoroughly* tested for toxicology, an expensive and time consuming study in itself. Few combined laboratory and field studies have been carried out to assess *in toto* what the public are consuming, in the way of nutrients, additives, trace elements and chemicals, and such studies followed up by appropriate animal studies. This is an area of research that badly needs development.

Children today, more susceptible than any to propaganda, are eating an increasing amount of sweets, lollipops, crisps and refined carbohydrate foods (biscuits, white bread, cornflakes etc.). Every one of these foods is processed to a high degree. Protein denaturation, vitamin elimination and general processing procedures will take their toll on natural ingredients. The author is not aware of *any* laboratory study where such ingredients are fed *in toto* to animals over a long term, simulating *as close as possible a modern child's diet* where analysis of health and morbidity is carried out. Such needs to be done. Our children are otherwise at risk.

In an attempt to educate his pupils into what constituted good food, one schoolmaster carried out a rather horrifying experiment in America, which is perhaps worth reporting here. In Cooper Elementary School, Vallejo, California, two rats were bought and caged. Pepsi in one cage was fed on what the children liked best; soft drinks, hot dogs, potato chips, candy, cookies and pie. Pepsi's hair came out, her eyes and hair were dull, she had sore feet and diarrhoea and failed to gain weight normally. In the other cage Suzette was fed on milk products, meat and eggs, vegetables and fruit, bread and cereals. Her fur was soft and silky, her tail was smooth, her eyes were bright and her movements quick and alert. She gained weight. Reasons for the difference in appearance of the two rats were then explained to the children in terms of nutrients and vitamins and a valuable lesson learnt. Whatever the method used, there is plenty of scope for nutritional education amongst teenagers and school children at the present time. The large choice of foods that is presented to them by modern day food science does in no way ensure a good choice in purchase. But the biggest need is for *directed* research in the field of nutritional science.

It is not possible within the scope of this book to analyse all processing procedures. The field is vast and ever expanding, and there is a great deal of data to sift. A brief summary here follows of some of the more basic procedures and the vitamin losses that occur.[4, 23] Particular reference is made to ascorbic acid in the case of vegetables.

1. *Losses from food storage*

Vegetables, especially, when stored, lose nutritional value. A soft vegetable such as spinach can lose 50% of its ascorbic acid content in 24 hours. Losses are less if the vegetable is refrigerated. Potatoes lose 20% of vitamin C in two months, 50% in five months.

2. *Blanching*

In the preservation of vegetables by canning, freezing or dehydration blanching is a basic first step. Involving immersion in hot water or steam, this process has a destructive effect upon water soluble vitamin C and B1. An estimated 10-30% loss of ascorbic acid occurs on steam blanching, up to 50% on water blanching.

3. *Deep freezing*

Losses vary with depth of temperature reached and time in storage. At −20°C spinach can sustain 55% loss of ascorbic acid, cauliflower 50% and beans 30%. Deep freezing procedures are superior to canning if blanching and cooking time are kept to a minimum.

4. *Canning*

At 65°F and storage for 24 months, 10-15% loss of ascorbic acid occurs in a vegetable. In hot climates the loss is 20-50%, and can be even greater for thiamine.

24

5. *Freeze drying*
10-20% loss of ascorbic acid occurs in fruits and up to 30% loss of thiamine. Losses of niacin and riboflavin are slight.

6. *Air dehydration*
Ascorbic acid is very vulnerable in this process and may be destroyed up to 100%. 50% loss of ascorbic acid is average. Other vitamins are fairly well maintained.

7. *Pasteurization of milk*
This process introduced for the purpose of destroying the tubercle bacillus (and brucellosis organism) also destroys certain enzymes in milk; the amylase, lipase, peroxidase, phosphatases etc. This enables it to store longer. Lost also are about 20% of ascorbic acid, 3-20% of thiamine. Niacin and riboflavin are hardly affected. Vitamins A and D vary more with time of year than with pasteurisation.

8. *Evaporation of milk*
This process affects protein quality in milk. 40% of thiamine and 60% of pyridoxine is lost also.

9. *Cereal refining*
The heat treatment of cereals in the preparation of breakfast foods has a detrimental effect on the protein (the lysine content) and Morgan and King[16,17] have shown this to affect growth of rats.

10. *Frozen meats*
Quick freezing can involve the meat in little nutrient loss. However the thawing of the meat is a more vulnerable procedure, thiamine, niacin and riboflavin being lost to a degree in the procedure. Precooked frozen poultry can involve losses of up to 40% thiamine.

11. *Institutional feeding*
Careless home cooking can destroy as many nutrients as institutional cooking but on the whole the latter is more detri-

25

mental to quality. Peppler and Cremer[18] give an analysis of household and canteen food losses:

Vegetable	*Vitamin B1 losses in* % Household	Canteen	*Vitamin C losses in* % Household	Canteen
Cabbage	49	62	57—67	82—85
Red cabbage	45	55	65	74
Pea soup	27	36	—	—
Mixed vegetables	56	54—63	—	—
Spinach	34	49	66	87

Institutional cooking can destroy up to 90% of the Vitamin C content of the potato (see Tables 2.1 & 2.2), through such procedures as soaking before peeling and precooking.

Platt, Eddy and Pellett[19] in their now historic study of hospital food show how lack of planning and lack of good cooking in hospitals can ruin most foods. Their report is not irrelevant even today when many complaints are heard regarding hospital meals. It is difficult to cater for any large number of persons and we have still much to learn in this respect. Would that more fresh food and raw food was served in an appetising fashion in hospitals.

12. *Irradiation*

To the author the most sinister of processing measures to be ushered in over the last ten years concerns irradiation of food. Great developments are expected in this field over the next 30 years. Irradiation pasteurises, sterilises, disinfects, disinfestates, and inhibits enzymatic processes such as sprouting. It is therefore a food scientist's ideal. In one simple easy measure, food can be sterilised and its storage life prolonged for a very long period. Irradiation inactivates all forms of bacteria, fungi, spores and insects and food can be treated while packed. It thus has huge economic advantages. The pressures are equally huge to introduce it. But is irradiated food healthy food? What else is killed in the foodstuff besides enzymes? Is it safe to eat?

There are basically three dangers to consider:
    (i)   Destruction of vitamins within the food.
    (ii) A mutagenic chromosome-damaging effect of the food.
    (iii) The formation of toxic substances in the food.

(i) *Vitamin destruction*

Vitamins A, B, C, E and K are particularly radiation sensitive[11]. Vitamin A is destroyed to the extent of 40% (carotenoids)

TABLE 2.1
Ascorbic acid content of potatoes at harvest (October), 5 and 8 months later, and in various states of preparation.

Time of analysis	Content of ascorbic acid, by %		
	Raw	Cooked & mashed	As potato flakes
Harvest time	100	62	26.7
5 months later	39	27	10
8 months later	35	22	9

Source: Bring S.V., Grassl C., Hofstrand J. T., Willard M. J., *J.Amer. Diet. Ass.*, 1963, 42: 320. Bring S.V., Raab F.P., *J. Amer. Diet. Ass.*, 1964, 45: 149.

TABLE 2.2
Percentage content of ascorbic acid in potatoes after various preparations.

Method of preparation	No of minutes allowed to stand after preparation			
	30	45	60	75
Potatoes steamed in skins	100	100		
Potatoes baked in skins	66	41		
French fried potatoes	66	50		
Potatoes peeled, cut and baked	52			
Potatoes peeled, steamed and mashed	37	36		5
Potatoes peeled, soaked and baked	24		11	

Source: Kahn R. M., Halliday E. G., *J. Amer. Diet. Ass.* 1944. 20, 220.

70% (vitamin A content). B is destroyed to the extent of 60 - 67% in beef, 68% in haddock, 87% in ham. Vitamin C is destroyed to the extent of 63 - 81% in strawberries, 4 - 26% in orange juice, 71.5% in asparagus, 86% in broccoli and 92% green beans.

Vitamin E is very sensitive to irradiation, a normal dose for whole milk destroying 61% of vitamin E. Natural vitamin K is less sensitive than synthetic. All the above figures are taken from the *Report of the Working Party on the Irradiation of Food* brought out by the Ministry of Health in 1964[21], and are vitamin losses in food that result from radiation at levels 'suited' to that food. Other B vitamins and vitamin D do not seem to be so susceptible to destruction.

Some protection from these losses can be enlisted by freezing the food or irradiating in the absence of oxygen but both these techniques add cost and are not likely to be carried out unless enforced by regulation. Handling food is a competitive business and expensive.

Such loss of vitamins cannot be ignored. There is a grave danger that in modern times the sum total of vitamin and nutrient intake will get *less and less* as more of these foods are eaten. These figures above are taken from reliable sources and they are large quantities — 92% losses, 81%, 86% etc. — not quantities that one can ignore.

Official sources tend to minimise the significance of these possible deficiencies:

> In assessing the probable pharmacological effects of continuous administration of irradiated foods to man or animals . . . it must be remembered that a mixed spectrum of foods, raw and processed, would be more than adequate to prevent the development of specific physiological aberrations in man[11].

In effect this means that man will keep good health *if* he eats raw foods and a good varied diet. Who eats raw food? Not so many of us and it is likely that less will do so as this century advances. Amongst teenagers, who set our future fashions, it is shown, later in the book, that few eat raw salads or raw fruit. The previous chapter has emphasised the large increase in sales of quick frozen vegetables. There is no reason to believe this trend will go into reverse.

The point is further brought home by the British Committee report on Irradiation[21]. Again vitamin loss is noted and in paragraphs 24 and 25 instances are given of *complete loss of thiamine when cooking was carried out on irradiated foods.* The U.S. Armed

Forces[25] carried out experiments to show that cooking irradiated foods caused further loss of vitamins and Witt et al.[26] found that thiamine was excessively lost when cooking followed irradiation. Animal experiments however failed to show pathology resulting from this[27].

Vigilance and caution will obviously be required when such techniques of food preservation as irradiation are introduced into general use. Commerce tends to coerce governments to introduce measures agreeable to financial interests and it takes the strong mindedness of a few individuals generally to stand out against such pressure; for vitamin loss is not the only hazard associated with irradiation, although perhaps the most certain one.

(ii) *Mutagenic damage*

The radiation levels in food that remain after irradiation are small. However, a potential hazard for man could present from the introduction into the body of extra radiation however small. There is still much controversy over this particular hazard and many consider it non-existent. The experiments that suggest any danger are of an uncertain nature.

Rinehart and Ratty[22] demonstrated a small increase in sex-linked recessive lethality in Drosophila fruit fly grown on food irradiated with heavy doses of X- or γ-rays. Holsten et al.[6] found that heavy doses of X- or γ-irradiation (2 Mrad) to sucrose, in which carrot cells were growing, resulted in the formation of cytotoxic growth inhibitory substances. It is postulated that these cytotoxic substances might affect the germ cells of those who ate such sucrose and their chromosomal structure be affected thereby producing such effects as congenital malformations and abortions in offspring. However both these experiments were conducted in very artificial environments and it is impossible to draw general conclusions from them.

Other scientists would heavily criticise such work and its relevancy and point out in defence that animals fed with irradiated foods over several generations have shown no ill effects. Goldblith[7] has pointed out that a 2-year feeding study on mice has been carried out where radiation sterilised pineapple, jam, sweet potatoes and fruit were fed at 35% dietary level with no ill effects noted. Other feeding tests with dogs, rats, chickens and pigs have shown no abnormality and have been carried out over 2 generations[1].

Makinen et al.[13] had found that juice expressed from pineapple, γ-irradiated with 30-500 Krad, immediately after irradiation depressed the rate of mitosis of onion cells and increased the incidence of chromosomal breaks. After 8 days storage this effect wore off though not at the highest radiation levels.

J. Schubert and E. B. Sanders[23] have recently detected cytotoxic and carcinogenic substances in irradiated glucose. The toxic compounds produced by irradiation were unsaturated carbonyls, which caused chromosomal damage in vitro.

Lofroth[12] writing in *Nature* is of the opinion that any compound causing cytotoxic damage should be considered hazardous to any type of cell, including the human cell, and that remembering the thalidomide disaster it is our duty to exclude these substances from our environment. Such is a minority view amongst nutritionists and food scientists and may overstate the danger. But as with all chronic long term toxic effects no one can accurately assess the danger that might arise and particularly as it applies to human beings. The danger is there.

(iii)   *Formation of toxic substances in food*

It is well known that irradiation can bring about changes in food chemistry that can lead to changes in food taste, odour and nutritional value. At recommended dosage levels these are generally small and not especially important. There are possible exceptions to this.

Above a dosage level of 5 Mrad and at about 6 Mrad protein changes take place in food. The sulfur amino acids in milk are degraded[9]. Beef protein releases ammonia and various amines[2]. The sulfur amino acids in breaking down form high smelling products such as hydrogen sulphide and methyl disulphide, which result in 'off' taste and odour. With many foods a dose of up to 5 Mrad is required to ensure sterility, and off odour and taste can thus follow from this. γ-radiation of wheat however at the low level of 0.5 Mrad, to prevent sprouting, seems largely not to affect the constituents of this foodstuff. Enzymes surprisingly seem largely unaffected by radiation, at this level.

Fats and polyunsaturated fats in particular undergo changes of oxidation on irradiation that give rise to toxic products — such as peroxides and carbonyls[11]. Animal unsaturated fats are more susceptible than vegetable. At 5 Mrad, digestion and absorption of fats can be slightly reduced and destruction of vitamin E, and especially vitamin K, take place from the action of some of the toxic compounds. The net nutritive value to the consumer has been shown to be unaltered despite this. The overall destruction of vitamin K produces haemorrhaging in rats fed irradiated foods [15, 20]. Kraybill comments upon this finding:

> The vitamin K radiation damage and haemorrhagenicity observed in experimental animals, of course, has no relevance to man, since human dietaries are composed of high vitamin K containing components in raw leafy green vegetables and other foods[10, 11].

Again the onus of responsibility is thrown upon *raw vegetables* to maintain health in the face of vitamin K depletion!

Irradiation enables food to be stored for a very long period sterile and uncontaminated. It also destroys a high percentage of the vitamin content of food and despite the strong economic arguments behind its use should be introduced very cautiously into the country. The public cannot afford to lose a substantial amount of their vitamins from food at present nutritional ratings.

Summary

In summary it can be seen that food processing of any nature detracts from the overall nutritional quality of a food, but such processing is necessary for modern food distribution purposes and handling. The author does not wish to deny in any way the functional importance of food processing in the handling and distribution of food. It is of paramount importance. What is questioned is the obsession with such a process that has possessed our society. In private gardens and allotments throughout the country lies a huge untapped source of fresh vegetable supply. If sufficient encouragement and appropriate education was given in the right quarters this source could be used to the benefit of the Nation's health *and* economy. Another instance of practical economy and sound nutritional thinking that could be put into practice in the home would be the home baking of wholemeal bread. It is easy and unfortunately fashionable to scorn such suggestions. The author feels that the matter is of urgency and will be of greater urgency as this century progresses. These two activities outlined above would do more to regain the standards of health to be expected of a modern civilised nation than any other measure likely to be pro-

The food and health of western man
pounded by modern government. Time is running out and so is money. Food if subject either to the process of technology and refining or handling and distribution will always be an expensive item. It will become even more expensive in the years to come. Remedies are required now.

REFERENCES TO CHAPTER 2

1 Blood F. R., Darby W. J., Wright M. S., Elliott G. A., *Toxicol. Appl. Pharmacol.* 1966, 8: 235.
2 Burks R. E., Baker E. B., Clark P., Esslinger J., *J.Agr.Fd. Chem.* 1959, 7: 784.
3 Cremer H. D., *Nutritio et Dieta* 1965 Fasc. 7 p.36.
4 Harris R. S., von Loesecke H., *Nutritional Evaluation of Food Processing.* Wiley, N.Y. and London 1960.
5 Hollingworth D. F., *Freeze Drying of Foodstuffs.* ed. G. B. Cotson, D. B. Smith, Columbine Press, London 1963, p.149.
6 Holsten R. D., Sugii M., Steward F. C., *Nature* (Lond.) 1965, 208: 850.
7 Goldblith S. A., *Nature* (Lond.) 1966, 210: 433.
8 Griffiths U.K., *Scientific Mission* (*N. America*) *Report No.* 66/20, Washington D.C.
9 Kraybill H. F., Read M. S., Linder R. O., Harding R. S., *J. Allergy.* 1959, 30: 342
10 ——*FAO/IEAA Report of Brussels meeting on Irradiated foods* 1962, 44.
11 ——Whitehair L. A., *Ann. Rev. Pharmacol.* 1967, 7: 357.
12 Lofroth G., *Nature* (Lond.) 1966, 211: 302.
13 Makinen Y., Upadhya M. D., Brewbaker J. L., *Nature* (Lond.) 1967, 214: 413.
14 McClure F. J., Folk J. E., *J. Nutr.* 1955 55: 589.
15 Metta V. C., Mameesh M. S., Connor B., *Fed. Proc.* 1959, 18: 537.
16 Morgan A. F., *J. Biol. chem.* 1931, 90: 1771.
17 ——King F. B., *Proc. Soc. Exp. Biol. Med.* 1926, 23: 353.
18 Peppler E, Cremer H. D., *Dtsch. Med. J.* 1964, 15: 313.
19 Platt B. S., Eddy T. P. *Food in Hospitals* publ. Nuffield Provincial Hospitals Trust, London 1963.
20 Read M. S., *Proc. Int. conf. on preservation of foods by ionizing radiations* July 27, 1959. Wash. D.C. U.S. Atomic Energy commn., (cited H.M.S.O. Report p.62, 1964).
21 *Report of the working Party on the Irradiation of Food* H.M.S.O., London 1964.
22 Rinehart R. R., Ratty F. J., *Genetics* N.Y. 1965, 52: 1119.
23 Schubert J., Sanders E. B., *Nature* (Lond.) 1971 233: 199.
24 Somogyi J., *Nutritio et Dieta* 1965 Fasc. 7 p.1.
25 Thomas H. M., Calloway D. H., 1961 Report No. 2-61 Chicago. *Quartermaster Food contamin. Inst. for the Armed Forces.* (cited H.M.S.O. report p.58, 1964.)
26 Witt N. F., Kraybill H. F., Read M. S., Linder R. O., Worth R. S., 1958 (contract No DA-49-007-MD-549).
Progress report No. 10—Washington (cited H.M.S.O. Report p.58, 1964).

27 Witt N. F., Read M. S., Worth W. S., Trabosh H. M., 1959. *Progress Report No. 12—Washington* (cited H.M.S.O. Report p.58, 1964).

Three
Bread — white
or brown?

Emotions tend to run high on bread. One is either a wholemeal enthusiast or an avid white consumer and one stands firm by one's convictions on the subject. Indeed, take care the man who questions these convictions! Bread however does provide a convenient focus for discussing the loss of food value sustained by processing, the nutritional risks involved, and the stand taken on these issues by health food groups, and wholefood groups in general.

There is a nursery rhyme which nicely makes a point:

There was a jolly miller once
Lived by the river Dee,
He worked and sang from morn till night,
No lark more blithe than he.
And this the burden of his song
Forever used to be,
I care for nobody, no not I,
And nobody cares for me.

The miller in days gone by was fighting the hazards of poor harvest, doubtful storage facilities, damp, infestation and other risks and no doubt had to adulterate, colour and dilute his product. He had to eke out his supplies as best he could or go out of business, so such additions as alum and chalk were not unusual in the trade. Chalk is still used today, though for other reasons. However the miller earned a bad name for his endeavours which has not exactly cleared in the eyes of the health food enthusiast today.

The accusation has changed and now it rests upon the charge that the miller profits from selling a denatured, processed and deficient product to a gullible ignorant public and all for the

34

sake of easy milling and good profits.

How true is this?

Food needs to be processed so as to be distributed as has been explained. To store in bulk a product must have 'shelf life'. It must not go rancid, and wholewheat flour with a content of oil derived from the germ can go rancid. It is not so easy to handle in bulk as fine white refined flour. But fine white refined flour goes to make a fine white refined loaf, and here lies the crux of the problem. For the public by and large like the appearance of a white loaf and will pay for its value in this respect rather than its nutritional quality. Or so we are led to believe! So the miller is doubly tempted to refine his flour both for storage purposes and for appearance. Who would forgo such advantages?

No really accurate surveys have been done on public preference. However history makes a point. Since the time of the Egyptians white bread has been prized as a luxury article. Sieved through fine meshes of papyrus grass to remove the bran, the Egyptians produced a fine cream flour used for the more costly bakings. Such flour was cream rather than pure white for it contained the germ of the wheat seed. The Bible gives us references. Abraham commanded Sarah to knead bread. Lot made it as an unleavened loaf and in *Leviticus* we find a reference to the value of fine flour: 'He . . . shall bring for his offering the tenth part of an ephah of fine flour' (*Leviticus*: 5.11). The Greeks too regarded black bread as food of common use and even poverty. So much for status symbols, which still exist today.

This tendency can be said to have played into the miller's hands. With the introduction of roller steel mills in the 1870s a white flour could be produced devoid of germ, devoid of 'creaminess', which could bake even more easily into a standard uniform loaf. The death knell sounded for wholewheat bread. By judicious mixing of his hard and soft wheats a miller could now bake a 'fine' loaf, of 'bold springy' texture, 'light and airy' enough to appeal to an unsuspecting public, who would judge by appearance and be cajoled into accepting a producer's product.

Extracted from wholewheat was the outer aleurone layer with its rich mineral content (and vitamins) and gone was the wheat germ, the 'heart' of the grain. The wheat germ has the best quality protein of the grain and the concentration of vitamins that go to make wholewheat a fine food. These, the wheatings, the throwout

35

from this 'civilising' process, go to make food for pigs, while humans consume what is left over. Five million tons of wheat are milled in this country and of this 1.4 *million tons is discarded as offals and wheatings — in actual fact the most nutritious part.* Table 3.1 shows the difference between wholemeal and 70% extrac-

TABLE 3.1
Nutritional composition of wholemeal and 70%
enriched white bread

Nutrient	Wholemeal bread	White bread
	mg per 100 *g*	
Vitamins		
Thiamine	0.2	0.18†
Riboflavin	0.1	—
Nicotinic acid	3.5	1.7 †
Pyridoxine	0.5	0.15
Pantothenic acid*	0.8	0.34
Biotin*	0.007	0.0008
Folic acid*	0.026	0.014
Linoleic*	800	530
Tocopherol*	2.2	0.85
Minerals		
Sodium	466	515
Potassium	261	106
Calcium	26	92†
Magnesium	89	22.6
Manganese	2.4	0.3
Iron	2.8	1.8†
Copper	0.46	0.13
Phosphorus	240	81
Sulphur	81	77

Other minerals contained in whole wheat flour[15]:
   Arsenic, Iodine, Bromine, Cobalt, Lithium, Titanium,
   Nickel, Aluminium, Tin, Silver
* Figures taken from Kent-Jones D. W.[21] and Sinclair H. M.[36]
All other figures taken from McCance R. A. and Widdowson E. M., *The Composition of Foods,* H.M.S.O. 1960.
† Enriched.

tion bread. Table 3.2 shows the vitamin loss sustained in refining. There is an 84% loss in pyridoxine, 80% loss in thiamine, 100% loss in vitamin E, 77% loss in biotin, 77% loss in nicotinic acid,

68% loss in folic acid, 67% loss in riboflavin, and 50% loss in pantotenic acid. There is a 50% loss in potassium, 75% loss in magnesium, 85% loss in manganese, 50% loss in iron, and 70% loss in phosphorus. Apart from this the protein of refined flour is of inferior quality to wholemeal (Fig. 3.1).

Why is this? The wheat germ of the wheat grain contains the plumule and radicle of the new shoot and new root. This part of the grain is therefore the 'power house'. Round the plumule and

TABLE 3.2

Proportion of certain vitamins lost in the milling of 70% extraction flour

Pyridoxine	84	
Biotin	77	
Folic Acid	68	
Riboflavin	67	
Pantothenic Acid	50	
Thiamine	80	(40% after replacement)
Nicotinic Acid	77	(40% after replacement)
Vitamin E	100*	

* Vitamin E is lost through milling and destroyed by chlorine dioxide.

Source: Moran T., *Nutr. Abst. and Reviews* 1959, 29: 1.

radicle will be gathered the quality nutrients which go to aid growth. The starchy endosperm is merely a reserve of cheap energy food later to be drawn upon by the wheat shoot. There is a danger in all processing that the quality products in the natural food are eliminated or denatured. Vitamins tend to be sensitive to extracting procedures. Minerals are often leached out with trace elements, leaving in both cases an inferior product. To break into the structure of a natural foodstuff inevitably incurs the risk of losing the finer elements that are involved in that very structure. Bread refining is a good example of this procedure. It is too easy to sacrifice quality for economic comfort, and too often done.

Flour processing

Having milled his product the miller then adds improvers, bleachers and maturing agents to aid the baking qualities of his product. Chlorine dioxide, the most commonly used of these, 'improves' baking qualities by toughening the gluten so the gluten

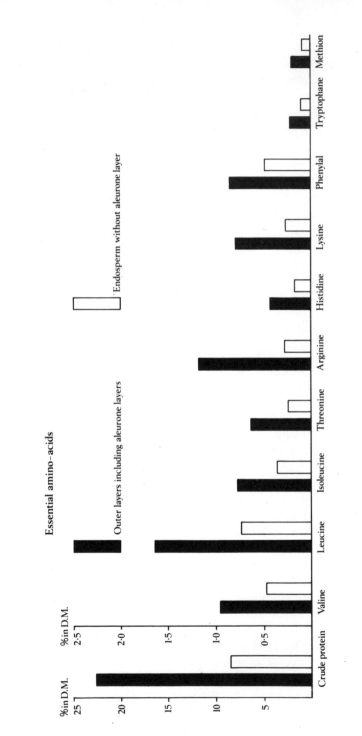

3.1. The difference in quality of protein between outer and inner layers of a grain of barley (from Schuphan W., *Nutritional Value in Crops and Plants*, Faber, London 1965

then holds better the gases of fermentation and maintains a good structure. A 'bold', 'airy', 'springy' loaf in modern baking parlance is the goal to be achieved. Standards however in this field are set more by appearance than by taste, and certainly take no account of nutrition. It is an interesting fact that French white breads are on the whole *not* produced with the aid of such improvers, and taste better.

Bread making is one more process to be industrialised as far as possible. How far is this justifiable? It is justified so long as our health does not suffer. By a fairly new process, the Chorley-wood process, dough is mechanically agitated at high speeds for a few minutes and fermentation time is reduced from two or three hours to a period of minutes, liquid ferments being added during the process. Chamberlain et al.[2] carried out certain tests on Chorley-wood bread and did not find that it had suffered nutritionally, but in what depth does one test for nutritional quality, and are chemical and laboratory tests ever sufficient? After all it is food for humans, not laboratory animals, and there is evidence that humans, quaint animals that they are, are rejecting this new tasteless product.

Kent-Jones in his *The Practice and Science of Bread Making*[20] allows himself to say that loss of flavour results from the Chorley-wood process, but in his view this is not important as a criticism, as bread is rarely eaten alone today or savoured for its taste!

The nutritional value of bread

Flour products contribute to our diet

27% of total caloric intake
26% of our protein
28% of our thiamine
27% of our iron (absorption is in question)
23% of our nicotinic acid
20% of our calcium
5% of our riboflavin.

Bread accounts for two-thirds of flour consumption, and is thus a significant foodstuff nutritionally, though consumption is falling. Consumption dropped from 51 oz per head per week in 1956 to 38 oz per head in 1966. Cakes and pastry consumption is however increasing a little to counter this.

Bread today is derived from 70% extraction flour and enriched with vitamin B1 (to a level of 0.24 mg per 100 g flour) nicotinic acid (to 1.6 mg per 100 g flour), iron (to 1.65 mg per 100 g) and calcium (to 235 mg per 100 g flour). In 1965[29] a strong case was put forward by an expert medical committee for the retention of a national flour of higher extraction rate in this country. The economic arguments put forward by the millers were too strong for this committee to withstand under the chairmanship of Sir Henry Cohen[34] and the doctors were overridden.

It is the contention of the author of this book *that the reinstitution of flour of extraction rate 95-100% would do more for the health of this country's people than any other single measure in the field of nutrition.* It would in addition be simple and cheap to introduce.

Proteins
The protein of wheat is not as biologically balanced in amino acids as certain animal proteins, such as milk and eggs. This is due to a low level of the amino acid lysine. Wholemeal bread is richer in lysine than refined white bread but at protein intakes common in the western countries this is no advantage. Our protein is varied enough to supply all amino acids. Chick[3], McCance and Widdowson[43], and McCarrison[27] have shown that refined flour is less effective in promoting growth of weanling rats than wholemeal, if the flour is the main source of protein. King et al.[22] fed white bread supplemented with lysine hydrochloride to underfed school children in Haiti and achieved increase in height, weight, skin thickness and haemoglobin (MCHC) compared to controls. McCance & Widdowson[43] however found that no advantage in height and weight gain resulted from eating wholemeal bread as compared to white bread in experiments in German orphanages. With bread contributing 18% of our protein in this country the advantage of the better protein served by wholemeal is lost and hardly relevant.

Vitamins
Extraction rates affect vitamin content considerably (Fig. 3.2). *Much of our supply of B vitamins is drawn from cereals,* including the lesser known vitamins, inositol and paraaminobenzoic acid. Table 3.2 shows the percentages of different vitamins lost from 70% flour. Wholemeal flour is seen to be a substantially richer source of all B vitamins than white flour which is seriously depleted

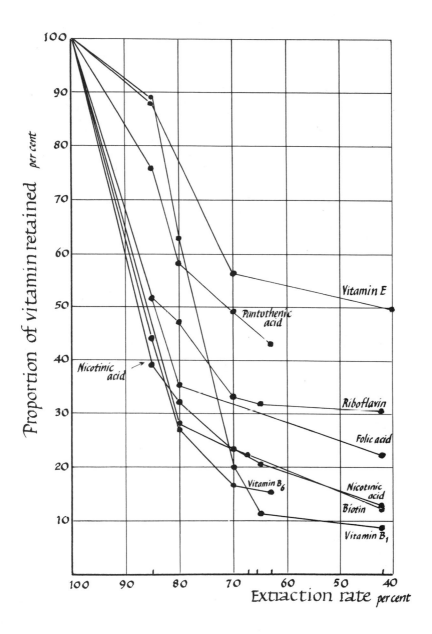

3.2 The relation between extraction rate and proportion of the total vitamins of the grain retained in flour (from Moran T., *Nutr. Abst. and Reviews*, 1959, 29:1–16)

in this respect. Accurate assessments of human requirements regarding many of these vitamins are lacking, while average intakes per head of population are available for but three of them (thiamine, nicotinic acid and riboflavin). Ignorance in fact is fairly substantial still as regards the place of many minor vitamins in human nutrition. Hence the care with which the medical committee in 1956 reviewed the nutritional position as regards bread and their reluctance to concede to the whiter flour[29]. Vitamin deficiencies are reviewed later in the book but a mention is made here of some of the relevant findings.

Adult requirements for thiamine are stated to be 0.4 mg per 1000 calories. Average intakes as estimated by current National Food Surveys range from 0.51 to 0.55 mg per 1000 calories. Riboflavin requirements are stated as being 0.6 mg per 1000 calories for the adult man. Average intakes range from 0.65 to 0.75 mg per 1000 calories. The group worst-fed at the lower end of the scale are adolescents living alone. Riboflavin intakes for this group can be stated to be just adequate, and often inadequate. Nicotinic acid requirements for the adult man are stated to be 4.0 mg per 1000 calories. Intakes for nicotinic acid range from 5.4mg per 1000 calories to 6.2 mg per 1000 calories in current National Food Surveys. Thomson[39] found in a large-scale survey of the diet of pregnant women in Aberdeen that 90% of women were taking in thiamine, riboflavin and nicotinic acid at adequate levels, as judged by the standards stated above. His estimated levels for nicotinic acid and thiamine intake were lower than the National Food Survey but still adequate. National Food Surveys record averages and recently it has been pointed out that we lack in this country an accurate survey of nutritional intake showing distribution differentials. An average is meaningless as it gives no indication of how many fall below the average and how many above. A sizeable number could and probably are suffering from subnutrition obscured in surveys by this averaging out process.

Folic acid deficiency on the other hand is now a common finding in pregnancy. Evidence presented in another chapter in this book points to findings that suggest that 30% of women suffer from folate deficiency in pregnancy and 3% suffer a macrocytic anaemia as a result. Folate, as its name implies, is found in leaves as well as in liver and the germ of cereals. The absence of green vegetables from the diet contributes as much to the presence of this nutritional deficiency in the population today as the eating of white bread, and probably more so.

Pyridoxine is another lesser-known B vitamin that also suffers depletion in the milling of flour. Sinclair[36] attached great importance to this deficiency in arguing against the national adoption of 70% flour in 1958. He regards the position as still hazardous and is concerned that our national intake of this vitamin is low as judged by American recommendations on intake. Pyridoxine acts as a coenzyme in the human body mainly in the metabolism of amino acids. It also probably acts on fatty acids enabling lengthening of the fatty acid chain to occur (e.g. linoleic to arachidonic acid). This last action may be relevant with regard to the fact noted by some that deficiency of the vitamin correlates with a raised blood cholesterol and the presence of atherosclerosis[13] though these are relatively unexplored fields. Richards[35] noted that in rats fed on 70% flour enriched with thiamine, (as our own flour) *pyridoxine deficiency was induced.* Thymus gland atrophy occurred, breeding performance deteriorated so markedly that scarcely any third generation animals existed and fits occurred prior to death of the young. All effects noted were corrected by the addition of pyridoxine to the feed. *No effects were seen on feeding 85% extraction flour, at which level breeding record was markedly superior.* Human beings are not rats but these experiments do raise important questions. They were accurately recorded and carefully reproduced on a large scale. There is therefore no reason to doubt that pyridoxine plays some important role in rat physiology. Secondly the thymus gland plays an exceedingly important role in human immunology. Many modern diseases are related to a break-down in immunological mechanisms. Could there be a connection therefore between deficiency of pyridoxine, accentuated under the conditions described by Richards (thiamine enrichment of low-grade flour), and auto-immune diseases?

The U.S. National Research Council (1964) tentatively suggested that daily pyridoxine requirements lay between 1.5 and 2.0 mg daily. Hollingsworth et al.[14] estimated pyridoxine intake in the country to range from 1.6 to 1.9 mg daily and this estimate was made before the refining of flour was authorised at the 70% level. It is thus likely that an intake lower than this is found in a certain segment of the population.

Many of the lesser known B vitamins are found in a wide

43

range of foods and in this fact there lies hope that deficiency is avoided. Pyridoxine itself is found in fruits, vegetables, meat, fish and milk as well as in cereals. Biotin is found in egg yolk, liver, fruit, milk and cereals. Pantothenic acid exists in meat, eggs, vegetables and cereals and Inositol is found in yeast, plants and grains. However any refining process destroys vitamins to an extent in a foodstuff and Schroeder in a paper in the *American Journal of Nutrition* shows how biotin, pyridoxine, and pantothenic acid are whittled away out of many foodstuffs in modern diets preparing the way for deficiencies.

Vitamin E is another vitamin destroyed in refined flour, and reference to the human requirements of this vitamin are made elsewhere in the book. The best dietary source in common use is wholemeal bread. Rich sources are found in some unsaturated oils. Butter, cheese, milk, meat and vegetables all contain a certain amount though often a small quantity. For a long time Vitamin E was not regarded as essential to man. The view on this is now changing and deficiency in humans recognised as a real entity. Vitamin E is all but totally destroyed in the refining of flour and in its maturing with chlorine dioxide.

Unsaturated fats are also present in wholemeal bread at a concentration higher than in refined white bread, though the latter does contain some of this fat which is mixed into the flour from the germ during milling. Some of the unsaturated fat in flour may be saturated by the chlorination that is involved in processing but even if lost by this means flour is not really a rich source of unsaturated fats. Flour provides only some 2 g out of a possible daily requirement of 14 g and the loss could be irrelevant.

To close this section, it is as well to remember that nutritional science is a young science and liable to serious modification of its views in years ahead. Requirements of lesser-known vitamins (and minerals) have not been quantified. Effects of marginal and sub-clinical deficiencies of vitamins have not been defined with regard to human health. Wholemeal bread is a rich source of B vitamins. The full value of the total B complex to health has not been valued as yet. It could be of considerable importance to man's health.

Minerals
The phytate bogey has haunted the steps of the wholemeal enthus-
44

iast for some years now and upset the equilibrium of he who maintains that wholemeal bread is superior to white bread in every respect. Some of the nutrients contained may be less available than at first appears. Wholemeal bread is richer in calcium, iron and other contained minerals than refined white flour but some of the calcium and iron forms an insoluble salt with phytic acid, also present in wholemeal flour, and the mineral is so rendered less available to the human body. In diets consisting for the most part of wholemeal bread a negative calcium balance can be induced by such intestinal interaction. McCance and Widdowson[24] showed this in 1942. Walker et al.[40] executing the same type of experiment though in fewer subjects queried McCance and Widdowson's conclusions as they found that adaptation in the human occurred over a long period. Taking wholemeal bread diets the calcium balance became positive after the *fifth week*. McCance[25] queried some aspects of Walker's paper but shifted his ground slightly in a reply at a later date and Widdowson[42] from experiments in Germany in 1951, which considerably extended the previous experiments, also modified her conclusions on the subject. Walker[41] summarised the position in a fairly complete review in 1951.

Taking into account the fact that bread now contributes but 15% of our calories and 13% of our calcium the sting has gone out of this particular controversy and its relevance is diminished. It is however worth making a few points. McCance and Widdowson[24] as well as others have definitely shown that a diet high in consumption of wholemeal bread is associated with binding of calcium in the gut and in some cases with the development of a negative calcium balance, *but* over a short period of time. The addition of calcium to wholemeal bread can rectify this position[43]. That the situation as regards calcium balance varies considerably and is inconsistent, is shown by Widdowson and Thrussell's[42] later experiments in Germany. Undernourished men and undernourished boys showed a range of calcium absorption and calcium balance on wholemeal bread that is confusing to say the least. Some of the men and boys concerned, on diets high in wholemeal bread, had a highly positive calcium balance and an absorption of calcium which reached 40 - 50% in some cases despite a daily consumption of 800 mg phytate!

The problem needs further research before understanding is complete. Many other factors have been shown to modify calcium

45

absorption besides the phytate content of bread. These include for instance the vitamin D content of the diet, the total calcium in the diet, the season of the year, the period of time the subject has been eating the particular diet, the magnesium and phosphorus content of the diet and the degree of malnutrition of the subject. The totality of the diet must also affect the intestinal flora. The flora in turn is known to hydrolyse phytate and thus influence the absorption of calcium. Very little work has been done on this particular factor and little can be stated as to the exact influence of the microflora in controlling mineral (and also vitamin) health. Breads themselves affect this balance[10] but details are lacking. It could well be that a diet high in vegetable and raw vegetable food produces quite a different floral 'effect' than one high in animal protein and refined foods and that this affects absorption of minerals and vitamins. Work has not been developed in this area of nutrition.

Other minerals besides calcium are present in wholemeal bread and in fact this bread is richer than refined white flour in phosphorus, magnesium, manganese, sulphur, copper, iron, potassium, lithium, boron and cobalt. Very little is known as regards the role of many of these minerals and trace elements in human physiology let alone their requirements. Deficiencies that result from a changing nutrition could be deficiencies of one or more trace elements but the study of these substances in food is undeveloped at the present time. Magnesium levels in wholemeal bread could give a significant nutritional superiority although workers in this field are not accurately certain of human requirements. Iron is bound by phytate in the gut in a similar fashion to calcium and the metabolism of calcium, iron, phosphates and phytates is interrelated in this respect. In fact it has been shown that iron absorption is more dependent upon calcium intake than upon phytate[33]. In the experiment upon orphanage children conducted by McCance and Widdowson[43] no significant correlation was found to exist between type of bread eaten and haemoglobin levels in the children, suggesting that bread, an inferior source of iron, provides this mineral equally whether in wholemeal or white refined form.

In summary the phytate content of wholemeal bread would seem to present a questionable and perhaps a small disadvantage with regard to calcium absorption. For him who eats such bread regularly, who does not rely upon it as the main source of calories,

46

who has a fair supply of calcium other than that contributed by bread and who takes a varied diet which contains vitamin D, there is no danger. Even without these conditions it has yet to be proved that intestinal adaptation does not occur. Concerning its other constituents wholemeal bread is a good source of other trace elements and minerals, and as such its consumption could provide a safeguard against possible deficiency of these elements, whilst further research in these particular fields is awaited.

Fibre

Fibre is a diminishing factor in our food. So much is obvious. Derived principally from foods such as raw fruits, raw vegetables and wholemeal bread, it can be seen that the increase in consumption of canned fruits, packeted, processed vegetables and refined flour foods will have contributed to a decrease in fibre content of food. Affluence tends to create a soft diet for these reasons. The intestinal contents as a result tend to bulk less and pass through the intestines at a slower rate. Such stasis produces its own complications.

Cleave and Campbell in their book *Diabetes, Coronary Thrombosis and the Saccharine Diseases*[4] attribute to the consumption of refined flour and sugar a number of our most important diseases today. (The subject is fully explored in Chapter 10 which deals with refined carbohydrates and disease). The consumption of refined flour products seems more directly implicated in the intestinal diseases (diverticulitis, haemorrhoids) and diseases associated (varicose veins, dental caries), while sugar *and* white flour consumption is associated in Cleave and Campbell's hypothesis with change of intestinal flora and such diseases as cholecystitis, appendicitis, pyelonephritis.

Dental caries is our most common degenerative disease! Soft sticky diets as well as sweet diets contribute to this. Sticky diets detract from tooth cleanliness and leave tooth debris. White flour products, and especially cakes and biscuits, are implicated. Rats fed dry powdered white bread showed only a marginally greater incidence of caries compared to those fed wholemeal bread[11]. Sucrose was shown in these experiments to be a more powerful cariogenic factor than bread. But a refined diet in general has been shown to increase caries, where white flour replaced wholemeal flour in the diet[37], and it is probable that both factors, sucrose and refining of foods, contribute to caries. Both contribute to cakes, biscuits, pastries and certain types of confectionery. Both no doubt contribute to caries and particularly so if the stickiness of the food is increased. Birch and Mumford[1] have shown that biscuit debris is singularly difficult to clean from the teeth.

Apart from these advantages concerning consistency, a separate factor has been identified in wholemeal bread that prevents caries[12]. Incubation experiments, in vitro, have shown that this factor protects dental enamel from demineralisation[19]. The factor is contained in the phosphate/phytate complex present in wholemeal bread.

Periodontal disease (disease of the gum and tooth supporting tissue) is as common as dental caries, and is another condition almost certainly linked to consumption of a soft refined diet.

Fibre, and the bran of wholemeal particularly, has been shown to markedly increase the passage of food through the bowel[5]. Bowel evacuations take place twice a day on a fibre-rich diet, not once, and the time the food lodges within the intestine is halved[5]. Whereas food might normally take 34 hours to pass through, with the bran of wholemeal this time is halved to 15 hours. Evacuation also is more complete. There would seem to be an important place for wholemeal bread in the prevention of disease, as also perhaps in the treatment.

Constipation and intestinal stasis have been the butt of many a joke. Professor McCance[26], a nutritionist and not a clinician, in his review of bread makes light of the subject and jokes over the concept that brown wholemeal bread is more healthy because it relieves constipation. The subject can often be treated humorously with good advantage and 'he who dwells upon his bowels is indeed not a likeable companion' but the jocularity can easily obscure what is probably a fundamental factor in health and disease. Cleave and Campbell[4] link intestinal stasis with the development of diverticulitis, haemorrhoids and more controversially, varicose veins. These three diseases contribute substantially to morbidity in this country, *and if only part of Cleave and Campbell's thesis were true and only a proportion of these diseases were prevented by the adding of fibre to the diet there would be still a saving of several million pounds to the Health Service and the freeing of many surgeons' time.* Humour could obscure an important truth. Fibre is more important as a nutritional factor than has so far been realised.

48

Additives in bread

I am the matron of an old people's home. I am very much interested in the feeding of the aged, and therefore encourage the consumption of brown, as opposed to white, bread in the belief that the former is of more value even though not comparable to 100% wholemeal.

Recently I noticed a greyish material gracing the dining room tables. On telephoning the baker to inquire the reason, imagine my feelings when a solicitous voice said. 'I am so sorry, matron; we have run out of colouring. It will however be added as soon as it comes in . . .'

I do not know whether I was the only mug left who didn't know of this double deception of the public but I do know that I am deeply concerned both from a moral and an alimentary viewpoint. . . .[38]

This letter was written to the *Sunday Express.* The colouring referred to in the above quotation was no doubt caramel. Other additives used in bread-making include[8] :

Bleaching and improving agents
Chlorine dioxide
Potassium bromate
Ammonium or Potassium persulphate
Benzoyl peroxide
Chlorine (cake flours)
Sulphur and dioxide (biscuits)
Emulsifying agents
Super glycerinated fats
Stearyl tartrate
Lecithin
Preservatives
Propionic acid
Calcium or sodium propionate
Acetic acid
Mono calcium phosphate

The Food Standards Committee Report on Bread and Flour[8] reviewed the position as regards additives in bread, their safety and their need, and cleared most of them, passing them as safe to use. Most concern has been expressed by the lay public over the

49

inclusion of chlorine dioxide in flour processing and it might be pertinent to outline a few of the toxicity tests that have been carried out on this particular improver.

Chlorine dioxide replaced agene (nitrogen trichloride) as principal improver in flour production in 1954. Sir Edward Mellanby[28] had recorded fits in dogs consuming agene in concentration higher than those found in bread but a toxic by-product could be identified in bread associated with the use of agene, and this improver was thus withdrawn from use.

Chlorine dioxide destroys the vitamin E content of flour[30] and can at high level interact with the essential lipids in flour to saturate the double bond[7]. At commercial levels of chlorine dioxide no toxic adverse effect has been shown.

Free chlorine used in the production of 'Angel' foods and layer cakes has a greater ability to saturate these fats but as the contribution of these lipids in cake to general nutrition is minute, no harm is brought about by such interaction.

In multigeneration experiments on rats, Hutchinson, Moran and Pace[17], in feeding flour at three times human consumption level, which had been treated with three times as much chloride dioxide as is normal, found no adverse effects in the health of rats. Impey and Moore[18] had found previously that growth rate had been retarded in rats fed the additive at concentrations of 30 ppm over four generations. This was an isolated finding in this field of research and not confirmed either by Frazer et al.[9] in thorough research on the substance in Birmingham or by tests on a variety of animals in America[32]. Dogs fed upon flour treated with 80 ppm of chloride dioxide remained in healthy condition for 13 weeks. Rabbits and monkeys on high concentrations grew well and remained healthy for 5 months and human subjects treated with high levels over a period of 6 weeks showed no adverse reaction[32].

Other additives in use include nitrogen peroxide which leaves traces of nitrite at concentrations of 3 ppm, benzoyl peroxide at 30 ppm which leaves residues of benzoic acid at 50 ppm; potassium bromate which leaves residues of 10 ppm potassium bromide, ammonium persulphate which can leave residues of 90 ppm ammonium sulphate, chlorine that is used in cake flour and which can leave residues of 4 ppm and sulphur dioxide in biscuits. The Food Standards Committee[8] reviewed the available evidence on these additives and concluded that no harm was evident from

50

their use. Mention was made, as is now usual in such circumstances, *that not enough evidence was available for full assessment of the chemicals under review.* Many of these compounds have been used in flour manufacture for 30-40 years. In previous years it was not customary to carry out full experimental laboratory tests on chemicals in food and many gaps in toxicology still exist as a result. It is hoped that both more money and more time can be devoted to it in the future.

Concern has been expressed by some that commercial interests influence nutritional interests[23] and mention has already been made of the fact, in the previous chapter. Leading nutritionists are often used in an advisory capacity to the food industry. They are naturally paid a salary for this essential service. Inevitably however their decisions in such delicate and intricate matters as toxicological assessments is affected by their allegiance to this industry. Not until the evidence or proof of toxic effect is strong or perhaps even overwhelming would they feel justified in stabbing their own industry in the back, or undermining its commercial success. This would be normal human behaviour in the circumstances. This situation is not made any easier by the fact that toxicological evidence is limited in extent and cases are generally of a borderline nature, and not clear cut. Far stricter independent control of such matters that effect public health therefore would seem to be justified. Independent bodies must judge these questions of health, and the men serving on these bodies must be uninfluenced by monetary gain. How else can one be objective in judging these more delicate issues.

Experiments in a German orphanage
In the final analysis it is not what a food contains that matters but how this food affects the health of man. Experiments on man are a necessity but have drawbacks. One of these drawbacks is that man takes many years to pass through one generation and long term study of man's health is therefore wearisome and drawn out. The long-term effect of refined flour consumption on man's health must therefore await final elucidation till many years are passed. Meanwhile Widdowson and McCance[43] in Germany after the last war, in conducting an eighteen month study in German orphanages, have attempted to assess the short term effects on health of eating different breads. The study is the only one of its

51

kind to have been carried out, unfortunately, and because of the great reliance that has been placed upon the results of the experiment, it is reviewed here. Widdowson and McCance in their summary are careful to point out that the conclusions drawn relate only to the conditions under which the experiment was carried out, and this particularly in view of the fact that the diet was so very different to what is eaten today in this country. In this respect the experimental diet might almost be described as peculiar and unique!

Three hundred and ten boys and girls were involved in the experiment from two orphanages, the children being grouped into five sections at one orphanage, three at another. The five relevant sections related to the type of bread eaten, the extraction rate of the flour varying from 70% to 100%. The children were split into five groups, eating:

100% wholemeal
85% bread
70% bread unenriched
70% bread enriched to 100% level
70% bread enriched to 85% level.

Enrichment involved the addition of thiamine, nicotinic acid, riboflavin, iron and calcium.

The diet of one orphanage consisted of 70% bread, 21% vegetable and 4% milk, by calorie intake. Almost total reliance was placed upon bread and carefully cooked vegetable to provide total nutrient intake. Vitamins A, D and C were given as supplements and Table 3.3 sets out the vitamin and mineral intake of the 70% unenriched bread group. They consumed healthy levels of all vitamins excepting riboflavin. No evidence of vitamin deficiency was evident and due to their high intake of vegetable it has been supposed that intestinal synthesis of the vitamin took place in these children. Fat intake is known to depress riboflavin synthesis and the Vohwinkel Orphanage taking in more fat showed lower excretory levels of this vitamin. Vegetables were conservatively cooked as soup. No cooking water was ever thrown away. Potatoes supplied 5% of calories. Bread intake for each group was unlimited preventing starvation from calorie restriction.

On this vegetarian regime all children grew very well and a striking improvement in general health was noted. Before the experiment the children had shown signs of under-nutrition. They

52

were then pot-bellied and had a certain amount of skin sepsis and hyperkeratosis; they were small for their age though lively and energetic. Height and weight improved throughout the experiment on all breads. Skin condition improved and freedom from infection

TABLE 3.3

Comparison of the nutrition of the children used in the experiment in German orphanages† with the nutrition of present-day large families in Britain.

Nutrient	Intake of nutrient per day	
	German children* in experiment	Families in Britain today**
Vitamins		
Vitamin A i.u.	2500 (2000)***	3410
Vitamin D i.u.	1100 (1000)	100
Vitamin C mg	150 (25)	37
Thiamine mg/1000 cals	0.6	0.52
Riboflavin mg/1000 cals	0.26	0.73
Nicotinic acid mg/1000 cals	6.8	5.4
Minerals		
Calcium mg	1150	860
Iron mg	9.8	10.8

* Children eating 70% unenriched white bread
** Families, social class C, D1 with 4 or more children
*** Figures in brackets denote amount of supplement given.
Source: Tables calculated from Widdowson and McCance[43] and *Annual Report of National Food Survey* 1966[16].
† Experiment conducted in post-war years by McCance R. A. and Widdowson, E. M. and reported in No. 287 of Special Report Series, Medical Research Council, 1954.

was noted. The wholemeal bread groups showed no distinct advantage over the refined white bread groups and the experiment showed that bread, white and wholemeal, supported by a diet of varied vegetable protein, with rich mineral and adequate vitamin intake, could support healthy growth in children.

When results of this experiment were published in Britain, bread companies took good advantage of the results and used the experiment for advertising their white breads. The scientists concerned were disappointed that such capital was made out of the work as the conditions of the experiment were in some respects unique and *not applicable to contemporary situations.*

Contemporary British diet is very different to what was consumed at these two orphanages, and great care is required before extrapolation of results is carried into our present day. Deficiencies in refined white bread have been outlined as deficiencies of fibre, vitamin B and mineral. However what is added to our present day diet may be of as much significance nutritionally as what is lacking. *We consume far more sugar, fat and prepared foods than was current at the time of the experiment.* White bread is consumed less and replaced by other forms of pastry, cake and biscuit food. Deficiencies of fibre, vitamin B and mineral take on a new significance in such a setting. To a considerable extent the orphanages covered their deficiencies of these three nutritive elements by a good intake of vegetables, both of the root and leaf variety. Their consumption of vegetables was higher than often found nowadays. All water in which vegetables were cooked was also saved, not an uncommon custom found to this day in Germany, and a custom which boosts mineral/trace element intake. By present-day standards their intake of vitamins C and D were very high and their intake of other nutrients very good (Table 3.3).

The experiment obviously needs repeating in a contemporary setting, though there is much doubt that over a short period it would reveal much in the way of evidence. The diseases that figure so greatly in present day society are diseases of chronic onset and experiments to reveal the nature of their onset would have to be run over thirty, not two years; a difficult problem.

Summary
The refining of flour to 70% extraction rate involves the following losses of nutrients from wholewheat flour:

Fibre	80%
Vitamin E	100%
Pyridoxine	84%
Thiamine	80%
Biotin	77%
Nicotinic acid	77%
Folic acid	68%
Riboflavin	67%

Pantothenic acid	50%
Manganese	85%
Magnesium	75%
Phosphorus	70%
Potassium	50%
Iron	50%

Trace elements: Lithium, Boron, Copper, Cobalt.

The effect of the loss of these nutrients upon the human body with regard to the refining of flour is not fully known. One thing is certain in this modern age of increased sophistication, nobody, and *certainly no child, can afford to throw away the above nutrients in the percentages shown.* The most important deficiency incurred by refining is probably that of *fibre.* To restore this alone to bread would probably in one simple stroke achieve more for the health of the whole nation than any other measure (see Chapter 10). But it would seem foolhardy also to ignore the other losses of nutrients concerning which there is so little information. Man needs the balance of vitamins, minerals and trace elements to live a full healthy life. For what reason should one deprive him of this right merely for the sake of economics, vested interests and commercial values? If but *one* deficiency was proved as caused by the refining of flour, for example folic acid, and this deficiency was found to cause ill health in the populace, as it does, then the government are in honour bound to reduce this balance. There are twenty and more other nutrients in bread.

REFERENCES TO CHAPTER 3

1 Birch R. H., Mumford J. M., *Dent. Practit. & Dent. Rec.* 1963, 13:182.
2 Chamberlain N., Collins T. H., Elton G. A. H., Hollingsworth D. T., Lisle D. B., Payne P. R., *Brit. J. Nutr.* 1966, 20:747.
3 Chick H., *Proc. Nutr. Soc.* (Lond.) 1958, 17:1.
4 Cleave T. L., Campbell G. D., *Diabetes, Coronary Thrombosis and the Saccharine Disease,* 2nd ed. John Wright, Bristol 1969.
5 Cowgill G. R., Anderson W. E., *J. Amer. Med. Ass.* 1932, 98:1866.
6 Cullumbine H., Basnayake V., Lemottee J., Wickramanayake T. W., *Brit. J. Nutr.* 1950, 4:101.
7 Daniels N. W. R., *Proc. Nutr. Soc.* (Lond.) 1966, 25.51.
8 *Food Standards Committee Report on Bread and Flour,* Min. Agric. Fish. Fd. H.M.S.O. 1960.
9 Frazer A. C., Hickman J. R., Sammons H. G., Sharratt M., *J. Sci. Fd. Agric.* 1956, 7:464.
10 Glatzel A., Hoffman K., *Nutritio et Dieta* 1961, 3:291.
11 Grenby T. H., *Brit. Dent. J.* 1966, 121:26.

The food and health of western man

12 ——*Arch. oral Biol.* 1967, 12:513.
13 Grozdova L. G., Paramanova E. G., Gorjachenkova E. V., Polyakova L. A. *Voprosy Pitaniya* 1966, 25.40.
14 Hollingsworth D. F., Vaughan M. C., Warnock G. M., *Proc. Nutr. Soc.* (Lond.) 1956, 15:XVii.
15 Horder Lord, Dodds C., Moran T., *Bread* Constable, London 1954, p.46.
16 *Household Food Consumption and Expenditure* 1966. Annual Report of National Food Survey Committee, H.M.S.O. 1968.
17 Hutchinson J. B., Moran T., Pace J., *J. Sci. Fd. Agric.* 1964, 10:725.
18 Impey S. G., Moore T., *Brit. Med. J.* 1961, 2:553.
19 Jenkins G. N., Forster M. G., Spiers R. L., Kleinberg I., *Brit. Dent. J.* 1959, 106:195.
20 Kent Jones D. W., Mitchell E. F., *The Practice and Science of Bread Making,* 3rd ed. Northern Publ. Co., Liverpool 1962.
21 ——*Proc. Nutr. Soc.* 1958, 17:38.
22 King K. W., Sebrell W. H., Severinghaus E. J., Storrick W. O., *Amer. J. clin. Nutr.* 1963, 12:36.
23 *The Lancet* 1956, 1:895.
24 McCance R. A., Widdowson E. M., *J. Physiol.* 1942, 101:44.
25 ——Widdowson E. M., *Brit. J. Nutr.* 1949, 2:401.
26 ——*The Lancet* 1955, 2:205.
27 McCarrison R. *Nutrition and Health* ed. Sinclair H. M., Faber, London 1953.
28 Mellanby E. *Brit. Med. J.* 1947, 2:288.
29 Memorandum of Med. Res. Counc. conf. on composition and nutritive value of flour. *The Lancet* 1956, 1:901.
30 Moran T., Pace J., McDermott E. E., *Nature* 1954, 174:449.
31 ——*Nutr. Abst. and Rev.* 1959. 29:1.
32 Newell G. H., Gershoff S. N., Suckle H. M., Gilson W. E., Erickson T. C., *Cereal chem.* 1949, 26:160.
33 *Nutrition Revs.* 1967, 25:218.
34 *Report of the Panel on Composition and Nutrative value of Flour* 1956, H.M.S.O., 1959.
35 Richards M. B., *Brit. J. Nutr.* 1949, 3:132.
36 Sinclair H. M., *Proc. Nutr. Soc.* (Lond.) 1958, 17:28.
37 Steinman R. R., Saunders M., Gilliland Y., Holub V., Tague C., *J. S. Calif. dent. Ass.* 1963, 31:400.
38 *Sunday Express,* letters, Sept. 8, 1968.
39 Thomson A. M., *Brit. J. Nutr.* 1959, 13:190.
40 Walker A. R. P., Fox F. W., Irving J. T., *Biochem J.* 1948, 42:452.
41 ——*The Lancet* 1951, 2:244.
42 Widdowson E. M., Thrussell L. A., 'Studies on undernutrition' *Spec. Rep. Ser. Med. Res. Council* 275, 1951.
43 ——McCance R. A. 'Studies on nutritive value of bread', *Spec. Rep. Ser. Med. Res. Council* 287, 1954.

Four

Infant and child nutrition

The extent to which children are affected by the changes in food habits so far outlined is now shown. There is malnutrition amongst our children and this derives from the sources already mentioned; the overconsumption of sugar, subsistence upon poor quality convenience foods and the lack of nutritional knowledge or understanding on the part of the mother.

The facts are as follows. They are derived from recent very thorough surveys in the nutritional field involving in most cases a large number of subjects.

33% of 450 infants examined between six months and two years are anemic.[9] Their haemoglobin levels are below 10gm per 100 mls. The equivalent figure in the United States is 44%![44]

59.6% of 261 infants examined at the age of six weeks are putting on weight at an abnormally fast rate and stand the danger of becoming obese.[52] These infants mostly artificially fed showed a weight gain velocity above the 90th percentile. Too much cereal feeding, sugar and prepared foods contribute to the diet.

33% of infants examined between the ages of one year and two years in a survey carried out in Scotland amongst 4,365 children were deficient in vitamin D intake. That is to say they were taking in less than 100 international units of vitamin D per day.[2]

The health of the mother contributes in large measure to the health of the baby born.

78% of 122 pregnant mothers in Newark, New Jersey, showed a hypovitaminemia at delivery assessed by maternal blood

57

levels.[19] Folate, thiamine and vitamin C were the predominant deficiencies.

59% of 200 households examined in the U.K. consume less than 30 mg vitamin C per head per day in the winter months, 20% during the entire year.[1] 30 mg of vitamin C a day is stated to be the marginal requirement. Over half the households in the U.K. in the winter months are in danger of taking in a deficient C intake.

25 to 30% of women suffer from folate depletion in pregnancy.[27, 57] They are found to have low levels of serum folate. Folic acid is a B vitamin found in liver, wholegrain cereals and green vegetables. It is easily destroyed by cooking.

Concerning preschool age, a Pilot Survey conducted by the Ministry of Health amongst 430 children revealed low intakes of calcium and vitamin D.[39] Calcium intakes only reached 60-80% of optimum requirements and vitamin D 25-60% of health requirements. Vitamin C intakes were only sufficient if welfare orange juice was taken. 52-59% of calorie intake was derived from bread, biscuits, cake and confectionery!

G. W. Lynch and S. de La Paz from the Department of Nutrition, University of London, in a survey of 4,382 school children throughout England and Wales found that 57% were involved in unsatisfactory feeding habits, 11% were classified in the 'extremely poor' category.[31]

In a previous study G. W. Lynch[30] showed that 25% of school children go without breakfast, or largely skimp their breakfast and rely upon snacks on the way to school. and school lunch to make up their nutrition. But the recent study by Bender et al.[4] shows that the school lunch itself is deficient.

Examining 772 school lunches in 48 schools in South England, Bender et al. found that the meals were insufficient in protein and energy value. Instead of providing the 33% of daily recommended intake of energy, they were contributing a mere 25%, in some cases 20%. There was heavy emphasis in most cases on sugar which provided in one startling case 33% of the total calorie content of the meal! The meals were heavy and lacking in fresh fruit and salad vegetables. Iron and calcium intakes were on the low side.

To underline the serious situation, Richardson and Lawson[43] comment upon the way our children eat in a letter to the *British*

Infant and child nutrition
Medical Journal. In a survey of 560 senior school children's eating habits it was shown that 41% of the children took school lunch, 31% bought food out of school instead, 20% brought food from home and 4% ate nothing at all! Those who bought food at tuck shops and cafés outside instead of school lunch mostly bought confectionery, low in protein and full of sugar and 'empty calories'.

Is this the way to bring up a generation? Is there ministerial or governmental concern over these figures? So far there is refusal to acknowledge that any problem exists. The health of our children it is reported, has never been so good. A child may appear large, fat and 'well fed', but this is not health. The large incidence of upper respiratory tract infections in childhood, the amount of fatigue reported by parents and the behavioural problems so commonly encountered could all derive from poor nutrition as well as other environmental factors.

The background picture
Other investigators have contributed to the picture we now have of infant and child health in this country, and it is as well to look at some of their findings.

The health of the pregnant mother must affect the health of the baby to be born. Perinatal mortality is correlated with poor physique, poor nutrition and low social class. Sir Dugald Baird[3] and Duncan et al.[15] surveyed perinatal mortality in Scotland before, during and after the last war. They were able to show that mortality increased as social class was lowered. A high mortality correlated with poor social conditions. Possible factors amongst the lower social classes causing this deterioration were lower standards of obstetrical care, poor nutrition and worse physique (shorter stature). However during the last war an abrupt fall in perinatal mortality was noted amongst these classes. At that time the nutritional standard of the poorer classes improved considerably. Rationing during the war evened out food supplies between classes, and priority foods were allowed to pregnant and nursing mothers. Luxury foods, butter and sugar, were eliminated for reasons of short supply and consumption of vegetables, potatoes, margarine and high extraction bread increased.[35] Duncan et al.[15] point out that no concomitant advance in obstetric care was apparent at the time, there being in fact a shortage of doctors. It is pointed out therefore that increased standards of nutrition amongst the lower classes during the war years resulted in improvements in perinatal health and decrease in mortality.

Studies from America[8], Australia[58] and Canada[16] carried out before and during the last war confirm the findings of Baird and Duncan et al. Perinatal mortality and incidence of prematurity both worsen as social class lowers, and the nutritional poverty of the lower classes is underlined as the factor causing this trend. Ebbs et al.[16] in their experiment in Toronto took a section of those on a 'poor' diet and supplemented the diet of this group with egg, orange, tomatoes, cheese, wheat germ, malt, iron and vitamin D. Compared to a control group obstetric complications and infant mortality dropped to a minimum in the treated patients.

Nutrition in pregnancy can also affect incidence of toxemia. Obesity predisposes towards toxemia[55, 56] as also does malnutrition and starvation.[58] 30 years ago toxemia correlated with undernutrition but nowadays to overnutrition. Obesity and poor quality diet lead to toxemia. A sound diet consisting of eggs, meat and liver (for protein), salad vegetables and fruit has been shown to prevent toxemia.[28, 50] Ebbs[16] fed a number of subjects eggs, milk, tomatoes, cheese, oranges, vitamin D and wheatgerm and reduced toxemia to very low levels.

There is probably a link also between certain congenital deformities and subnutrition. And it has recently been postulated that the high incidence of spina bifida in certain western countries is correlated with poor nutrition. Professor R. W. Smithells working from Leeds University on twin studies has detected an environmental cause as certain and a nutritional one as most likely in the aetiology of spina bifida.[49] Work is in process to identify the nutritional factor.

Pitt and Samson[40] in a retrospective study correlated spina bifida with low vitamin C intakes in pregnancy, cleft lip with low Bl, and congenital heart with low protein intake. However this retrospective type of study is prone to many inaccuracies and little store can be set by their findings. In a more interesting experiment Peer et al.[38] attempted to assess the place of vitamins in pregnancy as a prophylaxis against congenital defect. Mothers were chosen for experimentation whose first baby had suffered a cleft lip or palate deformity for it is known that in second pregnancy the likelihood of deformity in such cases is 5%. An attempt was made therefore at prevention. Supplementation with B and C vitamins in the first three months of second pregnancy achieved a 50% reduction in expected deformity, as well as reduction in other deformities presenting, compared to controls. In the Philadelphia Lying-in Hospitals, studies[25, 41] show that dietary counselling is as successful as vitamin supplementation in the prevention of deformities in the foetus and is basically a more sound approach.

Perhaps the most significant change in childhood nutrition over the past fifty years has been the change from breast to bottle feeding. The disappearance of breast feeding from the maternal scene and its replacement by the bottle has altered the pattern of infant feeding significantly. Solids are fed at an early age in the form of cereals, prepared infant purée foods and sugar. An intensive campaign of advertising has ensured the sale of these products and one brochure states that 'some babies do best if they are given solids from birth'. This is highly questionable advice in view of the findings of L. S. Taitz[52]. A high velocity of weight gain in the first months of life is *not* healthy and inevitably leads to obesity. The high sodium content of puree foods has been attacked as a danger in that it could predispose to hypertension.[10]

Artificially-fed infants have a higher incidence of upper respiratory tract infection and gastro-enteritis.[5] There are almost certainly some factors in breast milk apart from colostrum that protect the baby from these infections. Recently Bullen et al.[7] have identified an iron binding protein in breast milk named lacto ferrin that has the property of inhibiting the growth of E. coli bacteria, that would give breast milk an advantage in protecting against gastro-enteritis. Human milk also contains 2 to 3 times as much vitamin C as cow's milk, that in cow's milk being destroyed by pasteurization.

Hooper[24] has shown that obesity is far more common in artificially-fed infants who also have a higher incidence of infection. These are the principal differences that make this an inferior form of nutrition.

Rickets is another danger that has re-emerged as a definite health risk to the baby born and brought up in a large northern city. Glasgow and Manchester have found that rickets is not uncommon in their communities. Richards et al.[42] found 9% of young

61

children between 12 and 24 months in Glasgow showing radiological evidence of rickets. Rickets is a disease brought on by lack of open air, sunshine and the lack of vitamin D in the diet. Breast milk contains about twice as much vitamin D as cows' milk though both vary in their content according to the diet of mother or cow. A child that was fed on 2 pints of cow's milk a day would receive from 3-45 international units of vitamin D, and from 2 pints of breast milk would receive 4-100 units.[33] Breast feeding is now unpopular. In Arneil's survey only 10% of mothers were breast feeding beyond two months, and the infant is now dependent for his vitamin D supply upon proprietary dried milks and cereals. These mostly are fortified with vitamin D. Farex, Farlene, Twinpack, Ostermilk and Cow and Gate are all fortified foods but unfortunately the amount of vitamin D that is allowed to be added to these foods has been seriously curtailed of recent years. This is due to the fact that excessive vitamin D intake can occur and can lead to disease in certain conditions of hypersensitivity.

Dr. G. C. Arneil, an authority on the disease, reports over 100 cases of florid rickets presenting at the Royal Hospital for Sick Children in Glasgow over the last 13 years.[42] More white cases than coloured were reported contrary to popular belief. Stimulated by this finding to undertake a much wider survey, Arneil and his colleagues[2] carried out a dietary study of 4,365 Scottish infants in 1965 to find that a large number of children were receiving inadequate vitamin D, and in fact taking in less than 100 international units of the vitamin a day, one fourth of their recommended amount. The number of children at risk is worrying:

At 3 months	4.3%	Infants received less than 100 1.Units. vit. D
At 6 months	8.2%	,, ,,
At 1 year	24.8%	,, ,,
Between 1st and 2nd year	33%	,, ,,

The disease is easily remedied, by 500 1.U. of vitamin D, and should surely not be tolerated in this day and age. The reasons for its recurrence are various but fairly certain.

Rickets is a disease of the second year though it can occur before this. Children are now weaned off milk early and are taking solid food by the third month. By the twelfth month a child is often sharing the family's food. The foods that contain vitamin D are butter, eggs, herring, liver, mackerel and milk,[34] but none of these foods contains any considerable amount of the vitamin and the quantity in butter, eggs and milk varies very much with the season; low values being found in winter. 100 g of egg yolk contains about 200 units of vitamin D, whereas the same amount of halibut liver oil contains 60,000 units. If the fortified cereals are still being fed in the second year, this is an additional source of vitamin D. Cod liver oil, the richest source of vitamin D, is not popular and very few mothers persist in its use. There is thus another argument for education of the housewife in how to buy foods that are richest in vitamins, minerals and health giving properties, to prevent such a deficiency disease occurring.

Vitamin C depletion in infants and young children probably occurs more often than is realised. Higgins et al.[22] in carrying out a small survey in Oxford came across a number of children with very low C levels. Picking their cases from poor home backgrounds 5 out of 16 children examined were shown to have C levels in the blood below 0.15 mg per 100 ml. One child showed clinical scurvy.

On the whole the move towards feeding of solids earlier in infancy, which will include vegetables and fruit together with the present easy access to vitamin supplements, has prevented C deficiency and scurvy. However, there rests a danger of under-diagnosis and under-estimation. Not every child that comes to hospital with the complaint of failure to thrive, with or without painful swollen legs, is thought of as scurvy and the diagnosis can be missed.[20] Obvious signs of bleeding gums and purpura may not appear till later in time. Demers et al.[13] collected 87 cases in Canada and Grewar[20] comments upon the disease from America.

It is a particular quirk of human nature that we do not always eat what is good or right for us! Children dislike vegetables and prefer sweets! Vegetables provide vitamin C, minerals and trace elements, sweets provide nothing but sucrose and dental caries. Dierks et al.[14] found from a survey of 120 pre-school children in America that vegetables were the most unpopular dish of all, whilst meat, fruit and sweets were popular foods. In the child who did not care for fruit, vitamin C levels were found to be low. Lamb et al.[26] and Bryan and Lowenberg[6] report similar findings from young children. There is no doubt that vitamin C foods are often partaken of sparingly by children. Losses of the vitamin are common in cooking and processing which factor also contributes to a low intake. Allen, Brook and Broadbent[1] have shown how 20-50% of families in the U.K. at any one time are consuming marginal levels of vitamin C, a minority definitely consuming deficient qualities, and it is probable that many children are existing on low levels of this vitamin, and suffering as a consequence.

Iron deficiency is common in infants. Sturgeon[51] diagnosed the condition in 50% of infants from homes of good economic means. Some years ago in N.E. Scotland 42% of infants under 2 years were diagnosed by Davidson et al.[11] to be suffering from anemia, bearing a haemoglobin level of 10% below the accepted normal. Davis et al.[12] in a survey in London found 22.4% of white children were anemic and 53.5% of West Indian immigrant children. In Cincinnati, U.S.A., Guest and Brown[21] found 30% of infants to be deficient. The same proportion has been estimated in Oslo.[36] There seems agreement that poor families are, as usual, at greater risk from deficiency of this mineral and there seems a significant correlation between the anemia of the infant and that of the mother.[47] Those that are anemic are more susceptible to infection.[32] In the most recent analysis Burman[9] finds 30% of infants from Bristol had low haemoglobin levels, below 10G per 100 ml. Sephton Smith[46] regards the cause of the anemia as purely dietary and affected to a degree by the mother's haemoglobin state before delivery. A small and underweight baby is always at greater disadvantage than a larger baby. The iron stores are less in the smaller infant. The growth spurt in the first six months usually depletes the iron stores considerably and the haemoglobin falls only to pick up after the second year.[46] Plasma iron levels are low at this time and iron binding capacity high, showing deficiency.

Foods which supply iron are meat, eggs, green vegetable and to a lesser extent bread. Meat is a rich source and Schulz and Smith[45] have shown the iron to be absorbed from meat four times more efficiently than egg and ten times more efficiently than from vegetables. Elwood[17] finds bread iron is absorbed inefficiently though ordinary enriched cereals can be a good source.[46] Fresh vegetables are undervalued and underused as a source of iron both for mother and baby. Vegetables and fruits can catalyse the absorption of iron from other iron rich foods eaten, and are valuable from this point of view.

Recommendations for the right approach to sound nutrition

for mother, infant and young child therefore rest upon certain fundamentals. For the mother, the three foods which should be the basis of a good diet should be:

(1) good protein
(2) fresh vegetable
(3) fruit

The carbohydrates and fat, the minerals and vitamins will look after themselves if these three foodstuffs form the basis of the diet. The good protein should include wholegrain cereals. For the baby breast milk is obviously best and weaning to take place slowly onto cereals, vegetables and fruit. Carrot juice and orange juice, naturally expressed in the home, are rich vitamin sources. Vitamin D can be supplied from the fresh air (if available!) or more certainly by means of a supplement. Definitely sugar should be curtailed in baby's food along with a ban on salt. There is no need for these two substances and their presence in the infant's diet is a menace.

School and teenage

The studies carried out by members of the Department of Nutrition, University of London, underline the need to rethink our policies towards nutrition of the schoolchild. Lynch and de La Paz found from a study of 4,382 schoolchilden in England and Wales that 57% were subject to unsatisfactory feeding habits.[31] In a previous study Lynch had shown that 25% of schoolchildren missed or skimped breakfast.[30] Taylor[54] had found in an earlier study that 8% went without breakfast and 38% had but bread and butter. Small breakfasts are invariably supplemented by snacks mid-morning and the school tuck shop or the local sweet shop comes into its own. It has been shown experimentally that a high protein breakfast is less likely to produce hunger cravings mid-morning.[37] Hodges and Krehl[23] in a study of 2000 teenagers in Iowa found the school lunch if taken was the most balanced meal of the day. However if not partaken of, it was replaced by chips, fizzy drink, candy and confectionery, occasionally a pie.

Bender et al.[4] as has already been mentioned, find serious deficiencies in school meals. Instead of providing 33% of calorie and protein intake, they are providing 20-25%. Richardson and Lawson[43] show how snacking is increasing amongst senior school children and lunch is omitted.

Taylor has attempted to assess the effect of this poor nutrition
65

upon health. Using a combination of oral and dermatological clinical signs, Taylor has attempted to assess health in relation to vitamin and mineral intakes. His approach is in some respects controversial but his findings are arresting. Because of this the Ministry of Health asked Dr. Taylor to examine 82 boys and girls between the ages of 11 and 13 years at a school in London. Doctors from the Ministry of Health and Ministry of Education were present. A summary of the findings is given in a report of the Food Education Society,[18] a private nutritional organisation. Taylor had found that 33% of the children had enlarged red fungiform papillae of the tongue, and 15% had fissuring of the tongue. Two children had tongues with some loss of epithelium and 2 had obvious cheilosis. These changes in the tongue are attributed to B vitamin deficiencies. Myoidema is a term Taylor has clarified to indicate loss of muscle tone in connection with B vitamin depletion.[53] Fifteen children were shown to have significant myoidema.

Another approach to nutritional study is that explored in a recent paper by Lynch and Oddy.[29] These authors attempt to assess the amount of poverty in the population and match this against calorie intakes as derived from National Food Survey reports. National Food Surveys are concerned with averages and it is always a speculation as to what range of values lies behind the average. One is concerned to know how far below the average certain segments of the population fall, and the number who are at risk from poor nutrition. In terms of quantity of people affected it would be enlightening to have the full range of data given in such reports so as to assess the reality of subnutrition. It is perhaps surprising that this has not been considered necessary up to the present time. Lynch and Oddy show a range of subnutrition unsuspected up till now.

Table 4.1 shows the number of children calculated to fall into families where there is but one wage earner and he or she earns £10 - £16 a week. Included in the table is the calorie value of the diet per head in such circumstances. About 630,000 children fall into the two lowest categories of nourishment. The inaccuracies and possible exaggerations of such measurements are counter-balanced by further considerations. Habitual patterns of food consumption, lack of nutritional knowledge, poor cooking facilities, poor housing conditions and lack of storage and refrigeration can all contribute to poor nutrient intake of the poverty section of the population. What is accessible and convenient is chosen in preference to what is nutritious. Cheap foods that 'fill the gap' are more often bought than the more expensive but better quality foods.

TABLE 4.1
Number of children living in families where the head of the household is the sole wage earner at a weekly income of between £10 and £16*. Calorie intake per head in such families**.

Children in family	% of families in this category	Total number of children in such families	Calorie value diet per head
1	37	272,320	2620
2	41	603,520	2340
3	12	264,960	2240
4	10	368,000	2000

* Source: Lynch G. W., Oddy D. J., *Med. Offr. Lond.* 1967, 117:353.

** Source: *Household Food Consumption & Expenditure for* 1966, Ministry of Agric. Fish. Food. 1968.

Bread, margarine, tea, packeted and tinned foods, cheap cakes and biscuits are eaten in quantity. Fruit, fresh vegetables and meat are more expensive and less accessible.

As Lynch and Oddy state, even assuming normal curves of distribution, the plight of children towards the lower end of the range could be serious. The father of the family will in most cases take the largest share of food available, the children next and the mother often the smallest. Variations found in individual requirements will inevitably mean under-nutrition and malnutrition are occurring in a segment of our present population.

The surveys outlined point to serious deficiencies in the school child's eating habits. Sweets, lollipops and crisps with the help of television advertising have eroded what innate good nutritional sense remained within the understanding of the average housewife and average family and the stage is set fair for widespread subnutrition. How far this will affect health in the long-term is hard to assess. Certainly obesity shortens life and elsewhere in this book have been listed the number of chronic illnesses that derive from the overconsumption of fats and refined carbohydrates. General fatigue and psychological disturbance in adolescence are no doubt the results of many environmental factors but nutrition should be included as a potent factor amongst these.

A most interesting experiment was carried out 'in the field' at two Salvation Army homes during and after the last war. The experiment was run by a Dr. Annie Cunning. The report written by Margaret Brady for a health journal is reproduced here, by her kind permission.

Coming nearer home, we have the illustration provided some years ago by two Salvation Army Homes. One was for children between the ages of three years and eleven years who were in need of care. Dr. Annie Cunning, who was deeply concerned with children's food and health, took a special interest in this Home, to which she was extremely generous. With the co-operation of the officer in charge, she arranged for modifications to be made to the children's diet. White bread was replaced by 100% whole-wheat bread (baked at the Home), savoury oatcakes replaced sweet biscuits, raw muesli often replaced cooked porridge, and black treacle replaced sugar. Salad, eggs and poultry were obtained from their own garden, and they had fruit instead of the usual sweet foods, and were given a good mixed raw salad each day, or rather twice a day. An important item in their diet was a drink called 'brose'.

Dr. Cunning was not a vegetarian, and the children still had meat as before.

The officer in charge of the Home thought it was all 'a bit of nonsense' to start with, but because of Dr. Cunning's interest and generosity—she had, for instance, given them lots of apples and a machine for grating vegetables—she willingly agreed to try the new diet. After six months she herself said that not only was the improvement in the children's health most marked, but that they seemed happier in themselves. This was particularly significant, for although, when they first came to the Home, the initial change of having regular meals and a loving and sympathetic and religious environment, would naturally produce certain good effects, there were clearly further improvements when the change of diet was made.

The second Home was for older girls from eleven to eighteen, who came from unsatisfactory environments or whose parents had, perhaps, gone to prison. Some of them were considered to be in a 'pre-delinquent' class — not actually in trouble, but living unhappily in situations where they were liable to get into difficulties with the authorities.

Following the success of the 'reformed' diet in the first Home, Dr. Cunning was allowed to initiate similar changes in the second. Again, the officer in charge was sceptical, but willing to try and after six months, she too was surprised at the changes in her girls. Not only were their complexions improved and their hair brighter, but she observed very notable improvements in their behaviour too. The girls became more co-operative, both with each other and with the staff, to whom they also became more responsive, as well as being more amenable to the essential discipline of the Home. They also became much better at organising and using their spare time happily and well.

It is not suggested, of course, that they all quickly and miraculously became models of good behaviour, but there was a remarkable improvement in their behaviour which was quite definitely related to the 'fresh, raw and whole' food that they were given.

Their daily salads were attractively set out on individual plates, and often included unusual items, such as sprouted wheat grain. In this Home, too, drinks of brose, which was strongly advocated by Dr. Cunning, were taken daily. The basis for brose is 1 tablespoon of 100% wholewheat flour or ground oats with half a teaspoon of sea salt, placed in a jug. One pint of boiling water was then added and the mixture was well stirred. To this could be added apple or orange peelings, as available, or a taste of black treacle, the brose being then allowed to cool. Some people add a little fruit juice too.

It has been shown that in rats[48] there is an optimum richness of dietary intake above and below which performance diminishes. Not only does growth slow, but reproductive performance diminishes and *voluntary activity* decreases. Are we producing sluggish teenagers by allowing slovenly eating habits, for in the end it is we who are responsible for our community? Who should curb advertising for confectionery? It is our own responsibility. The public are in the end responsible for themselves. The evidence is now available. It must be shown to the public and our true needs highlighted. Then change can be brought about by intelligent reappraisal of our children's requirements. The evidence is slowly accumulating that all is not well in this 'sugared' generation and that health does really derive from what we eat. This chapter has been at pains to point out that there are in large areas of the community infants and school children suffering from the effects of poor nutrition. There is an urgent need for reform.

REFERENCES TO CHAPTER 4

1 Allen R. J. L., Brook M., Broadbent S. R., *Brit. J. Nutr.* 1968, 22:555.
2 Arneil G. C., 'Dietary study of 4365 Scottish infants', *Scottish Health Service Studies No. 6*, Scottish Home & Health Dept., 1967.
3 Baird D., *J. Obst. Gyn. Brit. Comm.* 1945, 52:339.
4 Bender A. E., Magee P., Nash A. H., *Brit. Med. J.* 1972, 2:383.
5 "Breast feeding and artificial feeding', The Norrbotten Study. *Acta Paediatrica* 1959, 48: Suppl. 116.
6 Bryan M. S., Lowenberg M. E., *J. Amer. Diet. Ass.* 1958, 34:30.
7 Bullen J. J., Rogers H. J., Leigh L., *Brit. Med. J.* 1972, 1:69.
8 Burke B. S., Beal V. A., Kirkwood S. B., Stuart H. C., *Amer. J. Obst. Gyn.* 1943, 46:38.
9 Burman D., *Arch. Dis. Childhood* 1972, 47:261.
10 Dahl L. K., *Amer. J. Clin Nutr.* 1968, 21:787.
11 Davidson L. S. P., Donaldson G. M. M., Dyar M. J., Lindsay S. T., McSorley J. G., *Brit. Med. J.* 1942, 2:505.
12 Davis L. R., Martin R. H., Sarkany I., *Brit. Med. J.* 1960, 2:1426.
13 Demers P., Fraser D., Goldbloom R., Maclean R., *Can. Med. Ass. J.* 1965, 93:573.
14 Dierks E. C., Morse L. M., *J. Amer. Diet. Ass.* 1965, 47:292.
15 Duncan E. H. L., Baird D., Thomson A. M., *J. Obst. Gyn., Brit. Comm.* 1952, 29:183.
16 Ebbs J. H., Tisdall F. F., Scott W. A., *J. Nutr.* 1941, 22:515.
17 Elwood P. C, 'Iron in flour', *Reports on Public Health and Medical subj.* No. 117, H.M.S.O. 1968.

Infant and child nutrition

18 *Food Education Society News Bulletin,* June 1967. F.E.S., 160 Piccadilly, W.1.
19 Frank O., *Med. News Tribune,* June 19, 1970.
20 Grewar D., *Clin. Paed.* 1965, 4:82.
21 Guest G. M., Brown E. W., *Amer. J. Dis. Childhood* 1957, 93:486.
22 Higgins G., Smallpiece V., Wilkinson R. H., *Brit. Med. J.* 1962, 2:479.
23 Hodges R. E., Krehl W. A., *Amer. J. Clin. Nutr.* 1965, 17:200.
24 Hooper P. D., *Practitioner* 1965, 194:391.
25 Kasius R. V., Randall A., Tompkins W. T., Wiehl D. G., *Millbank Mem. Fund Quarterly* 1955, 33:230.
26 Lamb M. W., Ling B. C., *Child Develop.* 1946, 17:187.
27 Lowenstein L., Cantlie G., Remos O., Brunton L., *Canad. Med. Ass. J.* 1966, 95:797.
28 Luikhart R., *Amer. J. Obst. Gyn.* 1946, 52:428.
29 Lynch G. W., Oddy D. J., *Med. Officer* (Lond.) 1967, 117:353.
30 ——*Med. Officer* (Lond.) 1969, 121:41.
31 ——*New Scientist* July 1, 1971, 51:32.
32 Mackay H. M. M., *Spec. Rep. Ser. Med. Res. Coun. Lond.* No. 157, 1931.
33 Macy I. G., Kelly H. J., Sloan R. E., *The Composition of Milk,* Nat. Res. Council publication 254, Washington D.C., 1953.
34 Manual of Nutrition, publ. Min. of Agric. Fish. Food, H.M.S.O. 1961.
35 Ministry of Food, *The Urban Working Class Household Diet,* 1940-1949, H.M.S.O. 1951.
36 Moe P. J., *Acta Paediatr.* (Uppsala) 1964, 53:423.
37 Ohlson M. A., Hart B. P., *J. Amer. Diet. Ass.* 1965, 47:282.
38 Peer L. A., Gordon A. W., Bernhard W. G., *Plastic Reconstruct. Surg.* 1964, 34:358.
39 *Pilot Survey of the Nutrition of Young Children,* 1963. Reports on Public Health and Medical Subjects No. 118, H.M.S.O. 1968.
40 Pitt D. B., Samson P. E., *Australasian Ann. Med.* 1961, 10:268.
41 Randall A., Randall J. P., Kasius R. V., Tomkins W. T., Wiehl D. E., *Millbank Mem. Fund Chart.* 1956, 34:321.
42 Richards I. D. G., Sweet E. M., Arneil E. C., *The Lancet* 1968, 1:803.
43 Richardson D. P., Lawson M., *Brit. Med. J.* 1972, 2:593.
44 Schulman I., *Jour. Amer. Med. Ass.* 1961, 175:118.
45 Schulz J., Smith N. J., *Amer. J. Dis. Child.* 1958, 95:109.
46 Sephton Smith R., *Arch. Dis. Child.* 1965, 40:343.
47 Sisson T. R. C., Lund C. J., *Amer. J. Dis. Child.* 1957, 94:525.
48 Slonaker J. E., *Amer. J. Physiol.* 1931, 96:547, 97:626, 98:266, 1935, 113:139, 1938, 123:526.
49 Smithells R. W., *Med. News Tribune,* July 10, 1970.
50 Stevenson R. B. C., *Med. Jour. Austral.* 1952, 1:317
51 Sturgeon P., *Paediatrics* 1954, 13:107.
52 Taitz L. S., *Brit. Med. J.* 1971, 1:315.
53 Taylor G. F., Chhuttani P. N., *Brit. Med. J.* 1949, 2:784.
54 ——*Brit. J. Ger. Prac.* 1967, 4:85.
55 Thomson A. M., Billewicz W. Z., *Proc. Nutr. Soc. Lond.* 1955 14:V, *Brit. Med. J.* 1957, 1:243
56 ——*Brit. J. Nutr.* 1959, 13:509.
57 Willoughby M. L. N., Jewel F. T., *Brit. Med. J.* 1966, 2:1568.
58 Woodhill J. M., Vanden Berg A S., Burke B. S., Stare F. J., *Amer. J. Obst. Gyn.* 1955, 70:987.

Five

Vitamin deficiencies today

I GENERAL

If the evidence so far presented in this book is true, then vitamin and mineral deficiencies must be appearing within the population. The next two chapters will analyse the extent to which they are manifesting. Overt or severe deficiencies are easy to type and diagnose. Subclinical or marginal deficiencies are more subtle altogether, and less certain to prove. That they exist however is shown by much of the following evidence. It is very likely that in the future more exact techniques will reveal far more of such pathology and enable the whole problem to be taken very seriously. For serious it is indeed if 50% of the population are suffering a deficiency, as has been suggested by a recent team working upon vitamin C. The upheavals in food technology and the food industry in general that are bound to increase in the future will call for greater vigilance than ever on the part of those safeguarding our health.

Vitamin A
There is no evidence on the whole for frank vitamin A deficiency in western civilized countries. Xeropthalmia, night blindness, ulceration of the cornea and skin lesions typical of vitamin A deficiency are rare in America and Britain. The eye lesions that occur in vitamin A deficiency develop from a drying of the conjunctiva. Roughness and wrinkling of this membrane produces a swelling and redness of the lids with resultant pain and photophobia. Softening of the cornea with ulceration may occur. Skin lesions and lesions of the mucus membrane also include papular

72

and pustular eruptions, a dryness, roughness and itching of the skin and keratinisation of the urinary tract.

Vitamin A is found in such foods as milk, butter, eggs, liver, fish and fish oils. Small amounts are found in ordinary meat and processed fish. Rich sources of the vitamin precursor carotene, are found in carrots, spinach, turnip tops, parsley and watercress; cabbage and lettuce being lesser reservoirs of this substance. Vitamin A deficiency is common in tropical countries as in South East Asia where the vegetable foods eaten are poor in carotene, and milk, butter, eggs and liver are not available.

Vitamin A requirements for the adult man are stated at 4000-5000 international units a day. From experiments conducted some years ago in Sheffield it would however appear that man can survive reasonably healthily on 1,300 units a day, 2,500 units a day providing a safe intake. In the experiments conducted by Hume and Krebs[51] in Sheffield in 1949, volunteers were put on an A deficient diet and observed over a period of months. When deficiency signs were clinically obvious, vitamin A was then fed at various levels to estimate the amount required to reduce signs of deficiency and restore blood levels. 1300 international units was found adequate for this purpose. Seven other volunteers fed 2500 units daily on a basic diet over a period of months developed no signs of deficiency and maintained adequate blood levels.

A reason for the large safety margin allowed for in setting daily requirements at 4000 to 5000 units is the fact that vegetables are not as efficient a source of the vitamin as fish or dairy foods and allowances are made for this fact. However consumption of eggs, butter and fish in western countries is such as to make deficiency of this vitamin unlikely.

Such would be the conclusion *but* for some recent research work from Canada reported by Hoppner et al.[44] This team examined the post mortem liver stores of a hundred Canadians of all ages and found that serious depletion was present in 32% of specimens. T. K. Murray[68] has since extended the survey to 500 autopsies. The autopsies studied covered a range of conditions and included both those who had died suddenly by accident and those who had died from specific disease. It is known that disease and especially febrile disease can depress liver stores of vitamin A and those who have died from such causes might be expected to have low liver content post mortem. However Hoppner and Murray found a suspiciously low liver content in many supposedly 'healthy' accident cases and query whether low vitamin A stores are not more common than is supposed amongst the population. 8% of all livers examined had no vitamin A stores detectable. 20% of post mortem livers in Montreal City were very depleted and 32% of all subjects (over 10 years of age) had low liver states (0-40 mg vitamin A per g).

A measure of difference was found between those who died from accident and those who died from disease. It is known that chronic disease states and fever depress A stores in the body and Hoppner records low liver A stores in patients who died from heart disease (111 mg per g) and even lower stores in those who died from cancer (55 mg per g). In the accidental death group the average vitamin A content for liver stores was 173 mg per g liver tissue, lower than previous studies.

Hoppner et al.[44] state that disease conditions, poor nutritional habits and other unknown environmental factors must have contributed to the low A status in such a high percentage of subjects. The point was made that a percentage of the normal population is either not eating the requisite amount of the appropriate food or is subject to chemical depletion of liver stores. Two possibilities cited by Murray[68] in this respect were cholesterol lowering drugs and D.D.T. Investigation was being carried out into D.D.T. levels in the body fat to assess whether a correlation existed with vitamin A stores.

Another possible reason for depressed vitamin A stores could be a high level of nitrite ingestion. Nitrite is used as a preservation in sausage, salami, and foods such as hot dogs, hamburgers and canned meats. Consumption of such foods is rising. The feeding of nitrite to animals can depress vitamin A stores in the liver[9] and the possibility exists that such interaction is occurring in the human.

In general, other dietary surveys indicate that vitamin A ingestion is adequate in the population. Further work is needed before the research findings of Hoppner et al.[44] and Murray[68] can be adequately explained. A situation analagous to that present with iron deficiency could be present also with vitamin A. A section of the population could be existing on low intake of this vitamin despite averages recorded in population surveys. Averages can be deceptive. A certain section of the population could feasibly

74

be at risk as regards vitamin A ingestion, and suffer liver depletion as a result. As with iron deficiency, stores can no doubt be depleted before blood levels fall.

Vitamin B1

The classical experiments of Williams, Mason, Wilder and Smith in 1940[89] in inducing thiamine deficiency in the human, showed the associated symptoms to be: fatigue, mental depression, generalised weakness, dizziness, backache, soreness of muscles, palpitation, dyspnoea and precordial distress (pseudo-angina), insomnia, anorexia, nausea, vomiting, loss of weight, atony of muscles, slight roughening of the skin, faint heart sounds, lowered blood pressure, bradycardia at rest, tachycardia and sinus arrythmia on exertion. In all cases physical activity was greatly decreased. Changes in the size of heart and oedema were not apparent in any case. No anemia, cheilosis or reddening of the tongue was noted.

Such a catalogue of symptoms is daunting! Not only are the symptoms of a general nature and often found associated with a multitude of other diseases but they are also of a type not easily measurable. How many doctors for instance would stop in their morning surgery to take blood for vitamin B1 assay on recording the symptoms of fatigue, even if thiamine deficiency presented itself as a possibility which is unlikely. Early diagnosis is difficult. Taylor and Chhuttani attempted to remedy the situation by devising a clinical test for purposes of measuring atony of muscles, one of the signs of thiamine deficiency. They named the condition diagnosed as myoidema, but controversy exists as to its significance, and few practise the test. There are no other tests of practical significance to aid in the early detection of B1 deficiency. Thiamine depletion or marginal thiamine depletion must therefore exist as a clinically indefinite state. Biochemical estimation of thiamine status is complicated and not a test usually performed by run-of-the-mill laboratories.

Beri-beri long associated with the condition is almost unknown in Britain. Moreover beri-beri did not occur in the experiments carried out by Williams, Mason, Wilder and Smith. Their human volunteers deprived of thiamine to the extent of taking a daily intake of less than 0.15 mg over a period of 88 to 147 days, recorded no symptoms of beri-beri. Oedema, cardiac dilatation and neuritic pain did not occur. Change in size of heart was not apparent. The authors therefore question the place of classical beri-beri in deficiency of thiamine and suggest this condition is the result of a multi-vitamin deficiency, not only thiamine. The list of symptoms catalogued by these research workers contains complaints which are for the most part subjective. The complaints however are common and everyday and should alert the physician to the possibility of thiamine depletion.

Recommended daily intake of thiamine by American and British standards is 0.4 mg per 1000 calories for the adult man. This is equivalent approximately to 1 mg intake a day. The volunteers in the experiment quoted above were taking less than 0.15 mg a day, approximately the amount of thiamine found in two slices of white bread. Thiamine is found principally in foods such as pork, ham, oatmeal, lentils, beans, wholewheat and soya flour. 36% of our thiamine intake is derived from cereals, 20% from meat and 20% from vegetables.[62] *Being water soluble, the vitamin is subject to loss from cooking, refrigeration and preservation.* Irradiation destroys it to an extent.

A daily intake of 0.4 mg per 1000 calories is by experiment more than sufficient. Some authorities[45, 53, 71] consider an amount half this in quantity, 0.2 mg per 1000 calories, as adequate, while others[28, 74] have stressed a need for a higher intake. Recent accurate research has defined an intake of 0.27 mg per 1000 calories as sufficient,[94] which with an intake of 2,800 calories would be equivalent to 0.75 mg a day.

It has been in dispute for some time as to whether high intakes of thiamine benefit health. Williams et al.[89] in their experiment already quoted found that daily intakes of up to 2 mg improved mental performance, alertness of mind, attentiveness and efficiency of physical performance. The work needs confirmation. Fat protects against thiamine deficiency and sucrose invokes it. A high fat diet can depress thiamine requirements considerably in the rat[4, 6, 7] while sucrose if fed to thiamine deficient rats will kill them![93] Additions of as little as 9% sucrose to the diets of these rats raised the mortality significantly.

Glucose and sucrose can induce in rats a thiamine deficiency more quickly than the feeding of more complex forms of carbohydrate such as potato starch, sorbitol or lactose.[69, 72, 73] The more complex carbohydrate forms are absorbed less quickly than sucrose and are therefore available lower in the intestine to feed intestinal flora and promote intestinal thiamine synthesis.[38] One can also say that the slower more gradual absorption of complex carbohydrate within the body stresses the metabolic reactions within the cell to a smaller degree.

Most of the population, as judged by National Food Surveys, take in at least 0.8 mg of thiamine daily. National Food Surveys record averages and do not show distribution curves. *There is therefore no means of estimating from such data the number of people existing on deficient intake.* Ziporin et al.[94] found that symptoms and signs did not occur until intake dropped to below 0.18 mg a day, a fairly low level. Signs of deficiency were then abolished when intake of the vitamin rose to 0.56 mg - 0.61 mg per day. In the study of cardiovascular health conducted by Cheraskin et al.[23] most adults were taking in more than 0.7 mg thiamine a day on dietary analysis. 5% were taking less than 0.6 mg. Brin[12] found that amongst the elderly dietary intake averaged 0.7 mg per day. Severe deficiency therefore appears rare. Most persons acquire an adequate intake even if classified as marginally adequate by some authorities. *However sucrose consumption is high and must obviously raise thiamine requirements* in the light of Yudkin's[93] and Gruber's[36] experiments with rats and pigeons. In school-children and teenagers it is quite conceivable that deficiency is induced by high sucrose consumption.

The refining of flour robs wholewheat of 80% of its thiamine, though refined milled flour has then by law to be made up to 0.24 mg per 100 mg in thiamine content. Refining cereals, and in particular rice, contributes to the prevalence of beri-beri disease in the Far East. In these countries rice can contribute 70% to the daily calorie intake and loss of thiamine can therefore be serious. In this country the loss of thiamine from flour certainly contributes to depletion of thiamine intake. It is less certain whether this causes disease.

More likely loss of thiamine in western countries could follow excess processing of food. In a previous chapter it has been emphasised how thiamine is susceptible to loss from irradiation, water treatment, heat treatment and refrigeration.[56] Processing if taken to an extreme could substantially reduce intake of this vitamin. Wholegrain cereals have a natural advantage in this respect in protecting against such possible situations.

It is apt to insert here a quotation from the book *Carbohydrate*

The food and health of western man

Metabolism by P. A. Soskin and A. G. Levine:[83]
It is only in recent years that the natural union
between vitamin B complex and carbohydrate which
exists in wholegrain and plants, has been broken by
the industrial processing of foods. Before this occurred
the supply of B vitamins was automatically adjusted
to the amount of carbohydrate eaten, so that the
occurrence of vitamin B deficiency with its consequent
disturbance in nutrition, is a comparatively recent
development in the western world.

Refining flour and the B vitamins
The major source of calories in this country (and America) are
flour and cereal products, sugar, potatoes and fats. They make up
approximately one fourth of the weight of the diet and about
80% or more of the calories. Refining of flour destroys a large

TABLE 5.1
Losses of vitamins in the refining of whole wheat

Nutrient	Wheat mg/g	Flour mg/g	Germ mg/g	Mill-feeds mg/g	Loss in flour %	Mill-feeds/flour, ratio
Thiamine*	3.5	0.8	22	17	77.1	21.1
Riboflavin*	1.5	0.3	5.5	4.2	80.0	14.0
Niacin*	50	9.5	80	150	80.8	15.8
Vitamin B	1.7	0.5	12	7.2	71.8	14.4
Pantothenic acid	10	5	25	22	50.0	4.4
Folacin	0.3	0.1	1.5	1.1	66.7	11.0
a-Tocopherol	16	2.2	125	38	86.3	17.25
Betaine	844	650	4,825	3,546	22.8	5.52
Choline	1,089	767	3,002	1,603	29.5	2.09
Gross energy kcal/g	4.4	4.3	5.1	4.7	2.3	1.09
Fat, %	1.61	0.87	8.03	3.7	46.0	4.25
Starch, %	57.21	68.66	18.05	22.13	+20.0	0.32
Protein, %	10.50	10.71	24.82	15.43	+ 2.0	1.44

Source: *The Millfeed Manual*, National Federation, Chicago 1967.
Moran T., *Nutrition Abstracts & Reviews* 1959, 29:1.

*Added back to refined flour to an extent. (Moran states that
77% Biotin also is lost through milling.)

percentage of B vitamins and it is conceivable that the loss of these nutrients significantly affects health. Table 5.1 shows losses sustained.

The significance of these losses cannot be properly assessed as so little is known concerning the complete physiological function of biotin, pyridoxine, inositol, pantothenic acid and niacin. If the populace are taking in marginal amounts of these vitamins, and it is probable that a certain percentage are, one cannot be certain at this stage of scientific advance what weaknesses will result. H. M. Sinclair[82] has for long maintained that the stripping of food of pyridoxine has contributed to atherosclerosis. Pyridoxine acts as a coenzyme in the human body mainly in the metabolism of amino-acids. It also acts on fatty acids facilitating lengthening of the fatty acid chain. Deficiency of pyridoxine has been correlated with raised blood cholesterol and atherosclerosis.[35] Richards[78] has noted that rats fed on 70% white flour develop pyridoxine deficiency and breeding performance deteriorated. Thymus gland atrophy was noted. Effects were reversed by the addition of pyridoxine. No effects were seen in rats fed 85% extraction flour. Thymus gland atrophy did not occur at this level.

Refining of many foods (cereal foods, canned vegetables, prepared potatoes, dairy products and canned meats) destroys pyridoxine so that refined sugar and fats contain virtually none of the vitamin. It is likely therefore that deficiency of this vitamin exists. School diets in America have been shown to be definitely short of this vitamin.[70] It has lately been shown too that oral contraceptives raise the requirements of pyridoxine within the body considerably.

Schroeder[79] also points to a dietary deficiency of pantothenic acid occurring in American and Western populations. In respect of pantothenic acid a level of 5.0 ppm was not reached in canned dairy products, canned root vegetables, legumes and frozen vegetables. Levels were also inadequate in breads and flours examined. It is probable that nutritional research over the next 20 years will uncover further facts regarding these deficiencies that result from the refining of foods. The whole complex of B vitamins are necessary for health. To strip food down and then replace one or two parts of the complex as a token gesture as it were is not wisdom. Neither is it physiological good sense.

79

Vitamin C

One can measure and diagnose scurvy and scurvy can be prevented by a low intake of vitamin C, as little as 3-5 mg in fact. Avoidance of scurvy however is not necessarily the only goal to be achieved. Ascorbic acid has other functions in the body besides maintenance of gum and tissue health. Scurvy might represent merely the end point in disintegration. It is a rare disease in this country, characterised by breakdown of mucus membrane and connective tissue. Bruising and haemorrhaging under the skin occurs and the gums bleed. Bone pains are common.

This is scurvy, a deficiency disease but vitamins do far more in the body than just prevent their deficiency. They are most of them catalysts in a wide range of biochemical functions within the human body, and are required for the full healthy working performance of this body. The difficulty has always been to assess how much vitamin is required for optimum performance. Interpretation of subtle physiological and psychological effects can lead to conflict.

Various techniques have been suggested and evolved for the evaluation of the optimum intake of ascorbic acid in man. Tissue vitamin C saturation can be measured. Biological indices such as optimum growth rate, reproductive viability, fertility, freedom from infection and disease can prove useful in animal experiments. Examination of tissue health can contribute from the assessment of wound healing and wound tensility. All these different measurements can give clues to vitamin requirement. The danger of such diverse assessment however is that the results also remain diverse and complex. Various vitamin C requirements are seen to suit various metabolic needs, and a final optimum requirement remains unproved. The problem in regard to assessment of ascorbic acid requirements is well and fully reviewed by Masek[66] and also by Sebrell and Harris[80] in their book *The Vitamins.*

Minimum C requirements for man have been cited at as low a figure as 3 mg per day ascorbic acid. This figure followed studies carried out by Abt et al.[1] on human volunteers, where vitamin balance was assessed by means of radioactive tracer work. Abt et al.[1] followed radioactively tagged ascorbic acid through the body, and measured urine and lung excretion of the vitamin, as well as total body stores and the half life of ascorbic acid. They found that balance could be achieved at the level of 3 mg per day. Earlier the

British Medical Research Council in 1944[13] had estimated minimum ascorbic acid requirements in the adult to lie in the neighbourhood of 5 mg a day. Scurvy was estimated as likely below intakes of 5 mg a day. Volunteers on 1 mg a day developed skin and mucosal haemorrhages after 26 weeks, gum changes and poor wound healing. Volunteers however on 10 mg a day were free of any symptoms. Moreover no difference in health was found to exist between the 10 mg group and another group taking 70 mg a day. The Medical Research Council therefore set their minimum requirement levels at 30 mg per day and later reduced them to 20 mg per day.

If tissue saturation, blood saturation or leucocyte saturation is a measure of optimum health, this saturation is achieved at an intake of between 50 and 100 mg a day ascorbic acid. Individual variations exist and blood levels fluctuate easily. Alternatively if one assumes that babies breast fed by healthy mothers are in optimum health, these babies average a blood level of 1 mg % ascorbic acid.[86] An adult intake of 80-100 mg would achieve this blood level. This could represent ideal intake.

Optimum growth in guinea pigs however is achieved at blood levels half this concentration, 0.5 mg per cent. Such blood concentration in the guinea pig also ensures maximum tensile strength of wounds, but not resistance to stress. Exposure to cold, physical stress, infection, pregnancy, sweating, muscular activity in animals increase ascorbic acid requirements for metabolic stress is intimately associated with vitamin C usage.[55] Experiments in man are less conclusive. Russian authors[92] favour the concept of stress increased ascorbic acid requirements and Russian dietary recommendations are therefore set higher than most other countries. Brozek and Grande[15] also quote work to show that intense mental activity and emotion raise requirements for ascorbic acid, and argue for high requirements on this basis. British workers are on the whole inclined to play down the stress component in vitamin C metabolism.

Extra high levels of intake in the guinea pig have been shown to increase the healing of an artificial wound[26] and have been shown to increase resistance against diphtheria toxin[54] as well as improve reproductive efficiency. Confirmatory results in man have not been forthcoming.

The British standard of 20 mg is set low. The American

standard of 75 mg is average. The Russian standard of 120 mg is high. Optimum ascorbic acid requirements in man if derived from saturation studies and guinea pig growth studies probably lie above 70 mg a day. The British Research Council's experiment was not designed to test health against stress or measure growth, but merely to record deficiency symptoms and it may well be that the recommended figure is for this reason set low. Proof that a higher figure for man is required for the maintenance of optimum health is hard to come by. It has been already shown that health in this respect is difficult to measure. More evidence is required and plenty of scope for research exists. Freedom from infection and resistance to disease are a measure of health. It would be interesting in this respect to ascertain whether the vitamin C status of the individual affects his susceptibility to disease. Vitamin C status and mental concentration also presents a field of possible exploration, suggested already by Russian experiments.

C Deficiency today

Scurvy is rare. It occurs in old people, and especially elderly bachelors and from time to time it appears in infants from impoverished homes. Scotland report more cases than England amongst the old and the majority of cases concern men who live alone. Thomson,[84] Brown[17] and Goldberg[34] report, altogether, some 200 cases collected over about 20 years. Diets of tea, bread and butter and canned foods are the cause of the disease in most cases.

Amongst healthy adults, blood levels of ascorbic acid are a fair indication of vitamin status. Blood levels decrease with age, and are lowered by smoking. Men have lower levels than women. Brook and Grimshaw[16] (see Table 5.2) found an average of 0.78 mg/100 ml in 20 year old men, 0.6 mg/100 ml in 40 year old men and 0.47 mg/100 ml in 60 year olds. Venulet[88] found sixty medical students averaged 0.6 - 0.9 mg/100 ml. Calder et al.[19] in a survey of 200 factory workers recorded ascorbic acid levels that ranged from 0.5 mg/100 ml to 0.9 mg (with an average of 0.78 mg/100 ml). Ages ranged from 16 to 63. From these surveys it would appear that the population range in blood vitamin levels lies between 0.5 to 0.9 mg per 100 ml. The lower levels would be sustained by the elderly and by those who smoke, the upper limits by those younger. It has been shown (see Table 5.2) by several

workers that smoking depresses the blood level of ascorbic
acid.[16, 19]

One survey from America is prominent by the number of
low ascorbic acid levels recorded. Setyaadmadja et al.[81] in a study
of 170 volunteers between the ages of 11 and 50 found 30% of the
group bearing an ascorbic acid level below 0.2 mg/100 ml and
55% below 0.5 mg/100 ml. Such low ranges are uncommonly
recorded.

Vitamin C intakes in Britain as assessed by the National Food
Survey reports annually, average out at about 50 mg of vitamin C

TABLE 5.2
Vitamin C blood levels as affected by smoking
and by age in 138 subjects

Non-smokers			Smokers		
Vitamin C plasma levels mg/100 ml			Vitamin C plasma levels mg/100 ml		
Age	Males	Females	Habit	Males	Females
20	0.78	1.06	Moderate	0.51	0.74
40	0.62	0.97	Moderate-heavy	0.44	0.74
60	0.47	0.75	Heavy	0.34	0.75

Source: Brook M., Grimshaw J. J.[15]

a day per head.[3] The limitation of these surveys and the deception
of an 'average' as a statistic where a range of distribution is concerned is shown up by Allen, Brook and Broadbent in the *British
Journal of Nutrition*.[2] In a careful analysis of the National Food
Survey reports and a survey they themselves carried out on 560
households, *it was found that as many as 54% of households in
the winter months were failing to achieve satisfactory vitamin C
intake* (30 mg per head per day). Throughout the whole year this
percentage came out at 25% (Fig. 5.1). They conclude that there
are no grounds for complacency over vitamin C intake in this
country, and a permanent percentage within the community are
consuming a deficient amount of vitamin C.

The food and health of western man

If we take 80 mg of vitamin C as a reasonable intake to ensure optimum health,[77] as assessed by animal studies, taking into account the role of this vitamin in preventing infection, restoring body tissue after trauma and achieving tissue saturation, then the majority of British people are deficient in this vital nutritional element (Fig. 5.1).

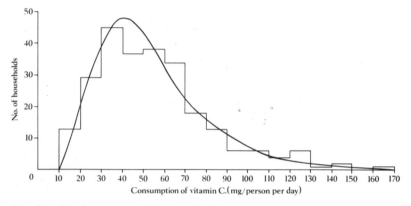

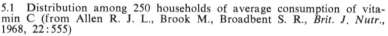

Consumption of vitamin C.(mg/person per day)

5.1 Distribution among 250 households of average consumption of vitamin C (from Allen R. J. L., Brook M., Broadbent S. R., *Brit. J. Nutr.*, 1968, 22:555)

Vitamin E

Vitamin E is elusive. Discovered 47 years ago by Evans and Bishop in 1922, no definite function and no definite physiological need has yet been ascribed to the vitamin as regards the human metabolism. In fact the vitamin has led medical research a 'will o' the wisp dance' over the 40 or so years since its discovery. Great therapeutic claims have at one time or another been associated with it and its absence in the diet has been named as causative in degenerative diseases, coronary thrombosis, infertility and many other conditions. Most of these associations do not stand the test of time, and most of the research defining E deficiency syndromes is inconclusive. Naturally the medical profession are suspicious of vitamin E and reluctant to concede a function to it as a result of this progressive disappointment.

Signs are now that the vitamin is finding its true place in human physiology. Its place in animal physiology in general has always been agreed.[11, 27, 60] Easier experimental conditions usually lead to clearer and quicker conclusions in animal research, the difficulty then being to relate findings to man. Vitamin E deficiency states in animals lead to a variety of conditions including sterility in male rats, foetal resorbtion in female rats, muscular dystrophy in rabbits and guinea pigs, encephalomalacia in chicks and haematological disorders in monkeys. The last of these findings is perhaps the most relevant to human physiology as indicated by recent research in man. Vitamin E deficiency occurs in man in cases of intestinal malabsorbtion and in infants following malnutrition. In such cases a haemolytic anemia has been found to occur similar to that produced experimentally in monkeys. Vitamin E deficiency can also be produced in premature infants fed a special milk rich in unsaturated fats. Haemolysis of the red cells occurs in this condition, confirmed by in-vitro tests with hydrogen peroxide, alongside anemia, oedema and thrombocytosis. Low blood levels of vitamin E occur which are correspondingly corrected by vitamin E administration. The haemolysis resolves under treatment. Vitamin E deficiency therefore does occur, under certain conditions, in man.

Vitamin E is found in a wide range of foods, though in small quantities in many.[18] The richer sources of the vitamin are vegetable oils (soybean oil, sunflower seed oil, safflower oil, wheat germ oil and margarine), some of the nuts (almond and walnut) and occasional vegetables (mature broccoli, outer leaves of cabbage and parsley). Wheat germ (Froment or Bemax) also contains a large amount of this vitamin. Fresh commercially cooked apple pie, fried fish and chips and any food that uses certain of the vegetable oils in cooking can contain a fair amount of vitamin E. Otherwise small sources are present in eggs, liver, butter, meat, tomatoes and peas. Average intake of the vitamin in America is 7.0 mg a day.[18] Consumption figures for this country do not exist.

Horwitt[46, 49] attempted to induce vitamin E deficiency in man. Feeding volunteers on a diet that included only 3 mg of vitamin E over a period of 5-8 years, changes were noted at the end of this period in the red blood cells. The cells proved less viable on testing. The red cell life was decreased, and haemolysis shown of the cells in vitro. Vitamin E therapy to the volunteers cured the phenomenon.

Serious disease states such as malabsorption in the adult[10, 14] and malnutrition in the infant[61, 65] can lead also to such haemolysis, as has already been mentioned, with anemia, oedema and thrombocytosis being recorded. A man suffering from the malabsorption syndrome over 6-12 months is likely to incur depleted plasma levels of vitamin E, lesions of smooth and striated muscle, and red cell haemolysis improved by vitamin E therapy. Infants with protein-calorie malnutrition in developing countries are also at risk of developing such an anemia.[61, 65] The decreased levels of serum protein in such infants are thought to play a part in the development of the deficiency. The protein in the blood is transport vehicle for the vitamin. Premature infants have also been shown to be at risk as regards E·deficiency, due to low maternal intake and low birth weight.[37, 75, 76]

The National Research Council in America state requirements as 10 to 30 mg of vitamin E a day. Using this measure 7% of Americans have deficient intake as estimated by Harris et al.[39] Estimates have not been carried out in this country.

Folic acid

Folic acid is a member of the B vitamin group and is found mainly in four foods; liver, kidney, wholewheat and green vegetables. Refined flour contains 32% the quantity of folic acid as wholewheat flour, for folic acid along with most other B vitamins is held most richly in the germ of the wheat. Vegetables are rich in folic acid and particularly lettuce, spinach, carrots, mushrooms, tomatoes, cauliflower and broccoli. Oranges also contain some of the vitamin though green vegetables are par excellence the source of supply for folic acid in our diet. If vegetables are eaten in small quantity responsibility for folic intake rests upon liver and kidney and these are hardly popular meats. Beef and pork do contain some of the vitamin but a 1/6 to 1/10 of the quantities found in spinach, as measured dry weight. Cow's milk has very small quantities, human milk being better supplied. Canned foods have a lower folic content than fresh and cooking can destroy some 40% of folic acid in food.

Folic acid is necessary in the body for the synthesis of essential nucleic acids, and is important in situations such as pregnancy where new tissue is growing fast. In pregnancy the demand for folic acid is raised, the body's stores are more readily depleted and in some cases produce megaloblastic anemia. That depletion of these stores and the anemia that often follows is so common is indicative of the questionable nutritional health of many mothers in America and Britain today. The situation might not be so important but for the obstetric complications that are associated with such an anemia.

Folic acid anemia in pregnancy

There is a fall in serum folic acid level throughout pregnancy.[5] In the normal woman vitamin levels at the end of pregnancy are half those found at the start. If the diet is insufficient or no supplements given some of these women will be definitely anemic, others deficient in folic acid.

Twenty-five to 30% of women will suffer substantial depletion of folate stores in a normal pregnancy. Beaven et al.,[8] Lowenstein et al.,[58] Turchetti et al.,[85] Lawrence and Klipstein[57] show a uniformity of finding in this respect. Willoughby and Jewel[90] found 33% of patients in Glasgow suffered subnormal postpartum serum folate levels and Lowenstein et al.[59] found that out of 311 pregnant women 50% showed low serum folate levels and 26% megaloblastic bone marrow changes. Using a less sensitive guide, the Figlu test, Hibbard[43] found 10% of a sample of 1480 women in Liverpool showed evidence of folic acid deficiency in pregnancy. Of course estimates of deficiency will vary with type of diagnostic method used in survey, the sensitivity of the particular method, and the moment during pregnancy that diagnosis is made. Megaloblastic anemia becomes more common as pregnancy advances and foetal demands increase. In Hibbard's large sample in Liverpool 5.4% of all pregnant women showed actual defective erythropoiesis in the marrow. Willoughby and Jewel[91] found 3.4% suffering from manifest megaloblastic anemia, Giles and Shuttleworth 2%.[32] If the figure then for incidence of folic acid anemia is taken as 2-5% and the figure for those suffering from depleted serum folate values is taken as 25%-30%, during pregnancy, an indication is then given of the severity of the situation and the extent to which it is found amongst the population.

Deficiency of folate in pregnancy is associated with accidental haemorrhage, abruptio placentae, abortion, foetal malformation, and premature labour. An increased risk of accidental haemorrhage was noted in megaloblastic anemia in pregnancy by Hourihane et al.,[50] confirmed by Coyle and Geoghegan[25] and Streiff and Little.[84]

87

In a study of abruptio placentae, Hibbard and Hibbard[42] showed low folate levels by a Figlu test in all but one of 73 cases. The relationship was confirmed by Hibbard[43] and again by Herbert.[40] An association was also found by Hibbard[43] between recurrent abortion and low folate levels, and also by Martin and Davis[63] while Martin et al.[64] successfully treated 15 cases of recurrent abortion by giving folic acid supplements. Foetal abnormalities[30, 43] and premature labour[31] have also been linked in aetiology to the deficiency of folic acid in the pregnant mother. It could be said with assurance that this vitamin is certainly not to be disregarded at time of pregnancy.

As to the main contributory cause of this anemia there seems little doubt that a *deficient diet is the most important one.* The parallel is with iron deficiency and in fact iron deficiency may indeed precipitate folate deficiency.[20] A body fed on a deficient diet just cannot stand the stress of pregnancy, and many diets that are taken today by pregnant mothers seem to be deficient in both iron and folic acid. Pregnancy will therefore precipitate anemia.

Reasonably accurate assessments of the amount of folate present in a normal diet have recently been made. Chanarin et al.[22] assayed 111 twenty-four hour food collections prepared for home consumption and found a mean folate content of 160 μg free folate. This compares with estimates made elsewhere that range from 157 μg to 193 μg.[24] The corresponding value for 10 daily estimations of a hospital diet was 117 μg.[22] Assays for iron showed 14.2 mg in the home diet, 11.3 mg in the hospital diet. Both diets are deficient in folate, the hospital diet is also deficient in iron. A man's needs are probably met by 50-75 μg of folate a day[41] while a pregnant woman needs a total of 250-300 μg of folate daily.[21] This increased need, as with iron, is just not met by the 'normal' diet. *Folate is lost in cooking and processing (up to 65%)* and most food is cooked or processed in some manner before eating.

Nutritional folate deficiency has occurred at times apart from pregnancy but there are generally environmental stresses that precipitate the anemia in such cases. In the woman lactation can do so.[67] A deficient diet can very quickly cause anemia at this stage. In a man, psychiatric depression, alcoholism, organic psychosis, as well as certain diseases such as rheumatoid arthritis and malabsorbtion can lead to a situation where a poor diet is taken and folate deficiency is induced. The elderly are also prone.

Foreshaw et al.[29] report on 17 such cases of nutritional megaloblastic anemia where diets of tea, bread and butter produce the disease. Some of the examples of daily intake and food eaten are worth quoting: 'tea, and milk and about three eggs a week'; 'tea, coffee, soup, potatoes and scones'; 'bread and milk because nothing else sticks down'; 'macaroni for lunch and sometimes a sandwich in the evening'. These were typical remarks passed by the patients concerned. Most patients in this group were suffering from depression, alcoholism or an organic disease such as peptic ulcer and hiatus hernia. These conditions obviously affected their food intake. Varadi and Elwis[87] report on an even larger group of nutritional megaloblastic anemias, indicating that the deficiency is perhaps more common than was thought previously.

Liver, wholemeal bread and above all fresh green and other vegetables are the sources of folic acid. Forshaw et al.[29] report a 37-year-old widow whose diet consisted of porridge, coffee, tea, soup, potatoes and a chop once a week who developed anemia. They record too the case of a 36-year-old man who drank and smoked, who ate macaroni cheese for lunch and a lettuce or a ham sandwich for supper, who also developed anemia. The small amount of lettuce, ham and white bread was just not sufficient to prevent anemia. Another woman reported in the survey relied upon a diet of tea, bread and butter and fried chips for her daily folate intake. Such foods as these recorded are all too commonly found as major components of food intake in Britain today. Sandwiches, chips, tea, bread and butter etc. are not foods that will prevent anemia. Snacks consumed by teenagers, elderly and the working man midday are often poor in folate content and should be remedied by intake of meat and fresh vegetables at some time during the day. Those who are partial to wholemeal bread have an advantage in this respect. Education is badly needed in this direction both for the sake of the pregnant mother and teenager. The elderly obviously need guidance as well.

It is worth finishing this section with a quotation taken from the report presented by C. Giles[33] on pregnancy folate deficiency in Staffordshire. The report covers a survey of 300 patients who had presented with megaloblastic anemia of pregnancy:

> Attempts to improve the diet of expectant mothers
> by repeated instruction in the antenatal clinic have
> met with only partial success for even in recent years

many patients gave a history of having taken a very poor diet throughout pregnancy, which included only 2 meat meals a week or less, few eggs and very little fresh fruit and vegetables.

Giles found 30% of his patients recorded this story of poor food intake as commented upon above. If our present economic depression increases and food prices rise in the future as they are doing at present, the situation will deteriorate. The outlook is on the whole very poor.

II IN THE ELDERLY

Old people often live alone, have usually little money to spend on food, suffer commonly from depression and almost always have false teeth! These are but four good reasons for an unsatisfactory nutrition. It is not surprising therefore to find that many surveys in recent years point to vitamin and mineral deficiencies existing in old age. It is questionable as to how far these findings are relevant with regard to the rest of the population. Old people are a separate social group with certain circumstances and customs peculiar to themselves. Many live in institutions such as old people's homes and hospital geriatric departments and suffer (or benefit) accordingly. Others often live in isolation in their own homes. Their deficiencies would seem to be related to their environment.

While acknowledging these facts it nevertheless remains true that a certain relevance exists to nutrition on a broader front. Old age is not an isolated happening and the deficiencies shown up at such a time might well have been set by the pattern of life in earlier years. Nutritional habits are deep ingrained and the weaknesses of such habits and the deficiencies inherent in them are exposed under stress. Old age might be considered as one such stress. Needs of the body change, availability of food lessens and infections and disease if present call upon nutritional reserves. An intake that is marginal and sufficient at 40 could become at 70 a deficiency.

The ageing body undergoes metabolic change. Its needs and

requirements alter. Both intake and absorption of nutrients declines. Blood vitamin levels will therefore be depressed as age advances. Part of this depression may be a natural phenomenon but part is also an environmental hazard. Decreased metabolic requirements can still be met under such conditions but stress of illness, trauma and infection cannot be met by such depleted reserves, and predispose to chronic illness and death. Rate of mortality relates in the old to vitamin C status and ingestion of less than 50 mg vitamin C a day has been correlated with an increase in mortality of 48% above average.[14] Recent evidence is presented from this country to confirm the relationship between vitamin C status in the elderly and mortality. T. S. Wilson[39] analysed the blood leucocyte vitamin C levels in 160 elderly patients admitted to a geriatric unit in Cornwall. One hundred and twenty-eight of the patients had buffy layer vitamin C levels of between 10-40 μg/10^8wbc with a mean of 22.2. Fifty had some form of psychiatric disturbance necessitating admission to the special psychogeriatric unit but the mean vitamin C level in that group did not differ significantly from the rest of the sample.

When the fate of these patients was studied, an interesting and rather startling fact emerged. Mortality among those with vitamin C levels of 12 μg or less was much higher than in those with levels of 25 μg or more. Forty-seven % of those admitted in the low vitamin C group were dead within four weeks compared with 25% in the high group — a difference which is statistically significant at the 1% level. Wilson is now carrying out a double blind study to assess the effect of vitamin C on mortality rate.

The old need less calories and less energy foods but it seems they need as much if not more *quality* in their food, that is to say vitamins and minerals. In animal experiments vitamin requirements seem to rise with age. Mills et al.[26] show that while 1 mg thiamine per kg food was adequate for rats of 11 months of age, 1.5 mg was inadequate at 18 months. In human subjects Rafsky and Newman[32] found lower levels of thiamine in the blood of elderly persons and lower urinary excretion on diets that *were considered adequate* for young people. Kirk and Chieffi[25] confirm this as also Dibble et al.[13] Andrews, Brook and Allen[3] found that elderly subjects took a lot longer than younger subjects to reach tissue saturation on 50 mg vitamin C.

If optimum health is to be sought for and achieved vitamin,

91

mineral and protein status in old people leaves much room for improvement. The frequent studies in the elderly that reveal deficiency of one type or another, some of which are quoted in this chapter, have brought to the attention of the public and the medical profession in the last five years the seriousness of the situation. The situation can be ignored and is ignored by those who consider that the old do not matter but the situation still remains. If people are living longer have they the right to live as healthily as possible or does infirmity rob them of this right? Geriatric medicine is unpopular but most of us one day will be geriatric ourselves. Its very unpopularity should make us wary of behaving negligently.

In most of the surveys quoted, estimations of deficiency are based on dietary analysis and biochemical estimation. Clinical science has not reached a stage where subclinical deficiencies can be accurately diagnosed by clinical examination, though Taylor[37, 40] and Brocklehurst et al.[9] are making an attempt to define criteria in this area of assessment. Signs of minor deficiency are not of an accuracy where lack of individual vitamins can be typed easily.

The most common deficiencies recorded in old age are, in order of frequency, those of vitamin C, iron, folic acid, vitamin D and vitamin B1.

Vitamins B1 and C

These two vitamins are water soluble, and they are therefore liable to heat destruction and water loss in cooking. Processing and refrigerating can also destroy them. Potatoes and vegetables supply most vitamin C to the elderly, and a certain amount of B1. Care therefore is required in how such vegetables are served. In institutions[30] and organisations such as 'meals on wheels'[15] much vitamin C is lost by large scale cooking and careless cooking. 70-90% can be lost from potatoes and vegetables at one level of cooking, 30-40% at another. Andrews and Brook[3] analysed the C content of food from four different sources; small and large welfare homes and small and large hospitals. Their results are shown in Table 5.3. Hospital vegetables had a much lower ascorbic acid content than those from welfare homes. Carrying out biochemical estimations of ascorbic acid status on patients from these different institutions, and comparing them to those living at home, lower values were found in the institutional subjects. Dietary intake of vitamin C for the institutional patients was estimated at below 30 mg a day. Kataria et al.[24] confirm these differences between patients in institutions and patients at home.

Fruit, the other food item that provides vitamin C is eaten less

TABLE 5.3

Vitamin levels in vegetables cooked in different sized hospital institutions

Vitamin C content of vegetables served at midday meals, as mg of ascorbic acid per 100 gm vegetable

Source	Boiled potatoes mashed, except†	Cabbage boiled	Brussels sprouts boiled	Swedes boiled
Small welfare home	7.3	—	—	14.0
Large welfare home	14.7†	—	16.5	
Small hospital	2.9	28.2	—	
Large hospital	1.2	11.1	—	
Hospitals sampled by Platt, Eddy and Pellett*	1.7	26.0	32.0	
% loss of vitamin	90	69	64	

Source: Andrews J., Brook M., Allen M. A., *Geront. Clin.* 1966 8:257

*Platt B. S., Eddy T. P. Pellett P. L., *Food in Hospitals.* Nuffield Provincial Hospitals Trust, Oxford Univ. Press, London 1963.

often than vegetables· for reasons of cost. Fruit is an expensive item for many old people but raw fruit is also seldom eaten for such reasons as 'it upsets my stomach' or 'my false teeth can't manage it'. It is not surprising then that intake of vitamin C is depleted in old age to low levels. O'Sullivan et al.[29] found 65% of a sample of old people were taking in less than 30 mg a day of vitamin C.

Indecision exists as to the optimum needs of old people but many workers in the field state that more not less vitamin C is

93

required to meet the demands of ageing, the stress of tissue breakdown, the likelihood of disease and infection. Morgan[28] puts these
requirements for vitamin C at 100-110 mg a day. Drake et al.[14] in
a survey of longevity find the mortality of old people ingesting
less than 50 mg vitamin C a day is 48% higher than the average
rating. In contrast those who took more than 50 mg vitamin C a
day had a mortality rating 20% lower than average.

Many workers have found low blood ascorbic acid levels in
old people. A fall with aging is 'normal' in that it is found in most
old people but how far the level should fall before being assessed
deficient is difficult to know. Different authors take different levels
as signifying deficiency with resulting discrepancy in results.

Calder et al.[10] in assessing several hundred factory workers
had arrived at average figures for blood ascorbic acid levels of
0.78 mg. per 100 ml plasma and for the leucocyte content, 26 μg per
10^8 cells. Kataria and Rao[24] comparing old people against these
average adult levels found those living at home average 0.49 mg/
100 ml and 26 μg/10^8 cells, those in hospital 0.18 mg/100 ml and
14 μg/10^8 cells. Those living in institutions carried the very low
figures of 0.09 mg ascorbic acid/100 ml plasma and 8 μg/10^8 cells
for a leucocyte count. Andrews and Brook[2] also found depleted
levels of leucocyte ascorbic acid in elderly people which correlated
in their survey with the presence of sublingual petechiae. Mean
levels in one group were 10.2 μg/10^8 cells and in the other 17.6 μg/
10^8 cells. Bowers and Kubik[7] using the less exact measurement of
plasma level found that 50 old people averaged 0.2 mg. ascorbic
acid/100 mls. plasma, and Batata et al.[5] measured 20% of geriatric
patients on admission to hospital as having a plasma content
below this 0.2 mg. mark and definitely deficient. Milne et al.[27] in a
survey of 500 men and women over 62 years of age in Edinburgh
found 50% of men and 58% of women were subject to vitamin C
intakes of below 30 mg. vitamin C a day, with correspondingly low
blood levels.

Griffiths et al.,[22] criteria unstated, estimated 41% of geriatric
hospital admissions as deficient in ascorbic acid and in a further
study,[22] using whole blood levels of the vitamin, 58% of admissions were stated as deficient. The same team in a further study,
this time headed by J. C. Brocklehurst[9] from Farnborough
Hospital, Bromley, found 77% of geriatric patients fell below 24 μg
ascorbic acid per 10^8 white cells.

This same team in this latter survey[9] attempted to correlate clinical signs of deficiency with vitamin blood levels, and at the same time carried out a double blind study with vitamins B1 and C. Cheilosis, angular stomatitis, nasolabial seborrhoea, glossitis of the tongue, hyperkeratosis of the skin and myoidema (not to be confused with myxoedema) were all found well distributed amongst the patients. Most of these clinical signs of deficiency responded well to therapy in the double blind study and a significant improvement in the general mental and physical condition of the treated patients was noted. Bed sores were improved. Such results would indicate that the stomatitis, cheilosis and other clinical symptoms and signs noted were due to vitamin B and C deficiency. It would also indicate that such symptoms are preventable. It was noted that many patients relapsed when treatment was stopped after a year and only a hospital diet given. Patients of this age in hospital have little desire to eat and suffer deficiency as a result, if trouble is not taken to make the food and environment attractive to them.

Vitamin B1 seems to follow vitamin C as regards the frequency with which the deficiency is diagnosed in old people. From dietary studies Brin[8] has shown 40% of one group of old people to be eating deficient amounts. Baker[4] confirms the low intake in a British study. Griffiths et al.[21] estimate some 59% of geriatric patients admitted to hospital as deficient in the vitamin and Brocklehurst et al.[9] in their more complete study find abnormally low thiamine activity in 61 patients in hospital out of 80 (76%). The clinical signs of deficiency noted by this team and commented on above were due to a combination of B and C vitamin deficiencies.

Folic acid
Folic acid is derived from green vegetables, liver and wheat germ. Folic acid deficiency, as measured by serum folate levels, is common in old people and has been found at frequencies of 15%,[38] 20%,[17] 30%,[33] and 40%.[23] Read et al.[33] in surveying 51 new entrants to an old people's home found 80% deficient in folate as opposed to 30% who lived at home. Dietary deficiency and not malabsorbtion has been named as the cause in surveys cited. Lack of interest in food leads to lowered intake and a poor quality diet. However supplementation with folic acid tablets can precipitate

95

pernicious anemia in the susceptible patient and dietary counselling is therefore a safer treatment. Megaloblastic anemia the consequence of severe folic acid deficiency is not common though it certainly occurs and is well recorded.[19] Dementia can also follow chronic folate deficiency.[36] Whether marginal deficiencies affect health and longevity, and whether old people can support a lower folate level than younger adults without incurring symptoms, is unknown.

Iron

If folic acid deficiency does not cause anemia as often as could be predicted from serum estimation, anemia as a result of iron deficiency is a known and proved hazard of old age. Goran et al.[18] found iron deficiency anemia present in 33% of old people and the incidence doubled amongst those living alone. Batata et al.[5] in a survey of 100 geriatric admissions in Oxford found a 33% incidence of lowered haemoglobin (below 11.7 g/100 ml) and a 10% incidence of frank hypochromic anemia. Davison[12] similarly estimates a 32% incidence of anemia in the elderly but in taking marrow specimens finds even more—75% as iron deficient. Powell et al.[31] found serum iron lowered in a third of geriatric admissions, with 50% admissions showing an iron saturation below 16%. Iron deficiency in old age is common.

Vitamin D

Old people also suffer from thin bones—skeletal rarefaction. It is in dispute as to how much this rarefaction is due to protein and hormone depletion (osteoporosis) and how much is due to mineral and vitamin depletion (osteomalacia). Both processes no doubt play a part as it has been shown that multiple deficiencies can exist in old people's diets. Calcium, phosphorus, vitamin D and protein can all be deficient in an old person's diet. Post menopausal hormone depletion contributes to the osteoporosis. A calcium intake below 500 mg a day and a vitamin D intake below 50 international units can lead to bony rarefaction. Exton Smith et al.[16] emphasise the place of vitamin D in the causation and treatment of this condition. Gough et al.[20] stress both calcium and vitamin D as important, while Smith and Harrison[35] in a recent study find that phosphorus, protein and vitamin D intakes all fall with age, that skeletal rarefaction increases with age but that a strong correlation does not exist between any one factor alone and clinical osteoporosis.

The frequency of rarefaction diagnosed in population and group surveys will depend closely upon the criteria of measurement used. It is difficult to standardise X-ray analysis. Estimates therefore vary from 8%[1] to 30%.[15] Beck and Norden[6] diagnose osteoporosis in 12% of males and 23% of females in a geriatric survey and Collins[11] finds an incidence of 8% in men and 18% in women.

Prevention and treatment
Opinions divide over the use that should be made of vitamin supplements in old age. The good clinician on the whole has an aversion to supplemental therapy. Rather would he attempt to correct the fault at source. Here however with regard to old people there arise difficulties. For reasons already outlined old folk lose interest in food and lose also their accessibility to good food. Dietary counselling can only hope to be minimally successful. More hopeful are attempts to improve social status and environment, to arrange for home helps to come in and cook meals for the old, to improve such services as 'meals on wheels' and to upgrade considerably the standard of food preparation and service found in large institutions. It seems obvious that in respect to certain vitamins institutional food is often of poor quality.

Having said this and recommended such changes it is still probable that the elderly will suffer deficiency, for appetite slackens and intake drops considerably with old age. One cannot be forced to eat and vitamin supplements may be necessary. Schulz and Kirsch[34] found appetite improved, mental and physical performance improved and serum proteins rose in a group of old people treated with a vitamin supplement. Brocklehurst et al.[9] recorded significant changes for the better in physical and mental health of the old treated with C and B1 supplements. Bed sores improved, and skin and mouth health improved in those so treated. It would thus seem that if a diagnosis of deficiency is made or suspected it is the responsibility of the doctor to correct this. This is most satisfactorily done in many cases by vitamin supplementation alongside social and dietary counselling. By such means one can attempt to make the last years of life a little more bearable.

Summary
As has been explained, accurate assay of vitamin deficiency in the population as a whole is awkward and difficult to make. Frank

vitamin deficiency presents as a separate clinical syndrome to subclinical or marginal deficiency and the latter is now accepted by most nutritionists as a reality. It is certainly a reality in the field of animal experimentation. Decrease in performance and activity, decreased resistance to disease, depressed fertility and longevity can all be shown at one time or another to result from marginal vitamin intakes. Appropriate experiments in man are difficult to undertake.

Evidence has been presented in this chapter to show that intakes of Vitamin B1 (thiamine), B6 (pyridoxine), Pantothenic acid, Folic acid and Vitamin C, are low and sometimes dangerously low in the population. Those who subsist on white flour products, poor quality vegetables, processed or poorly cooked, and little meat will be short of vitamin B intake. It is important also to mention again in this context the researches carried out by Yudkin and Gruber which showed in rats that glucose and sucrose ingestion can induce a thiamine deficiency much more easily than the ingestion of complex carbohydrates and starch. Sucrose once more presents as a nutritional menace. Most processing procedures will deplete food of thiamine. Refined flour is an example where the whole B complex is lost to a large extent in the processing procedure.

Regarding vitamin C, 54% of households in Britain in the winter fail to achieve satisfactory C intakes of 30 mg per head per day. Some authorities would consider this level in itself as deficient and not marginal. Smoking depresses vitamin C levels and the increasing replacement of fresh fruit by processed counterparts adds to the risk of deficiency. Vitamin C is an important vitamin and evidence points to its effect on increasing longevity, and affecting health over a fairly wide sphere.

The elderly for reasons stated are more at risk than other age groups. Low levels of B, C, and D have been found in many surveys. The situation is even more serious for those who are both poor and old.

Vitamin deficiency is common in western civilised countries presenting as explained in its subclinical marginal state. The rise in food prices and especially of meat, vegetables and fruit expected in the years ahead does not bode well for the future. The remedy is fairly simple. In the context of these two vitamins, B complex and C, it is to advocate the consumption daily of wholegrain cereals in place of refined white flour cereals and the daily

98

consumption of fresh fruit. The remedy is even pleasant as well
as being practical!

REFERENCES TO CHAPTER 5

I GENERAL

1 Abt A. F., von Schuching S., Enns T., *Amer. J. Clin. Nutr.* 1963, 12:21.
2 Allen R. J. L., Brook M., Broadbent S. R., *Brit. J. Nutr.* 1968, 22:555.
3 *Annual Report of National Food Survey Committee. Household Food Consumption and Expenditure* 1965, H.M.S.O. 1966.
4 Arnold A., Elvehjem C. A., *Amer. J. Physiol.* 1939, 126:289.
5 Ball E. W., Giles C., *J. Clin. Path.* 1964, 17:165.
6 Banerji G. G., *Biochem J.* 1940, 34:1329.
7 ——*Biochem J.* 1941, 35:1354.
8 Beaven G. H., Dixon G., White J. C., *Brit. J. Haematol.* 1960, 12:777.
9 Beeson W. M., *Fed. Proc.* 1965, 24:924.
10 Binder H. J., Spiro H. M., *Amer. J. Clin. Nutr.* 1967, 20:594.
11 Bird H. R., Culton T. G., *Proc. Soc. Exptl. Biol. Med.* 1940, 44:543.
12 Brin M., Schwarzkopf D. A., Davies D. A., *J. Amer. Ger. Soc.* 1964, 12:493.
13 *Brit. Med. Res. Council Spec. Rep.* Series 280 H.M.S.O., 1953.
14 *Brit. Med. J.* 1966, 1:935.
15 Brozek J., Grande F., *Abnormalities of Neural Function in the Presence of Inadequate Nutrition*, publ. Thomayer Coll. Prague 393 SFN, 1959.
16 Brook M., Grimshaw J. J., *Amer. J. Clin. Nutr.* 1968, 21:1254.
17 Brown A., *Glasgow Med. J.* 1951, 32:95.
18 Bunnell R. H., Keating J., Quaresimo A., Parman G. K., *Amer. J. Clin. Nutr.* 1965, 17:1
19 Calder J. H., Curtis R. C., Fore II., *Lancet* 1963, 1:556.
20 Chanarin I., Rothman D., Berry V., *Brit. Med. J.* 1965, 1:480.
21 ——Rothman D., Ward A., Perry J., *Brit. Med. J.* 1968, 1:390.
22 ——Rothman D., Perry J., Stratfull D., *Brit. Med. J.* 1968, 1:394.
23 Cheraskin E., Ringsdorf W. M., Setyaadmadja A. T. S. H., Barrett R. A., *Int. J. for Vit. Res.* 1967, 37:449.
24 Chung A. S. M., Pearson W. M., Darby W. J., Miller O. N., Goldsmith G. A., *Amer. J. Clin. Nutr.* 1961, 9:573.
25 Coyle C. V., Geoghegan F., *Proc. Roy. Soc. Med.* 1962, 55:764.
26 Danielli J. F., Fell H. B., Kolicek E., *Proc. Nutr. Soc. Lond.* 1946, 4:197.
27 Dinning J. S., *Rev. Can. Biol.* 1962, 21:501.
28 Elsom K. O'S., Reinhold J. G., Nicholson J. T. L., Chornock C., *Amer. J. Med. Sci.* 1942, 203:569.
29 Forshaw J., Moorhouse E. H., Harwood L., *The Lancet* 1964, 1:1004.
30 Fraser J. L., Watt H. J., *Amer. J. Obstet. Gynec.* 1964, 89:532.
31 Gatenby P. B. B., Little E. W., *Brit. Med. J.* 1960, 2:1111.
32 Giles C., Shuttleworth E. M., *The Lancet* 1958, 2:1341.
33 ——*J. Clin. Path.* 1960, 19:1.
34 Goldberg A., *Quart. J. Med.* 1963, 32:51.
35 Grozdova L. G., Paramanova E. G., Gorjachenkova E. V., Polyakova L. A. *Voprosy Pitaniya* 1966, 25:40.

The food and health of western man

36 Gruber M., *Nature* 1950, 166:78.
37 Gyorgy P., Cogan G., Rose C. S., *Proc. Soc. Exper. Biol. Med.* 1952, 79:446.
38 Haenel H., Ruttloff H., Ackermann H., *Biochem Z.,* 1959, 331:209.
39 Harris P. L., Hardenbrook E. G., Dean F. P., Cusack E. R., Jensen J. L., *Proc. Soc. Exper. Biol. Med.* 1965, 65:739.
40 Herbert V., *Tr. Assn. Amer. Phys.* 1962, 75:307.
41 ——*Arch. Intern. Med.* 1962, 110:649.
42 Hibbard B. M., Hibbard E. D., *Brit. Med. J.* 1963, 2:1430.
43 ——*J. Obstet. Gynec. Brit. Comm.* 1964, 71:529.
44 Hoppner K., Phillips W. E. J., Murray T. K., Campbell J. S., *Canad. Med. Ass.* 1968, 99:983.
45 Horwitt M. K., Liebert E., Kreisler O., Wittmann P., *N.R.C. Bull.* 1948, vol. 116.
46 ——*Amer. J. Clin. Nutr.* 1956, 4:408.
47 ——*Amer. J. Clin. Nutr.* 1960, 8:451.
48 ——*Borden's Rev. Nutr. Res.* 1961, 22:1.
49 ——*Vitamins & Hormones* 1962, 20:541.
50 Hourihane B., Coyle C. V., Drury M. I., *J. Irish Med. Ass.* 1960, 47:1.
51 Hume E. M., Krebs H. A., *Spec. Rep. Ser. Med. Res. Counc.* (Lond.) No. 264:1949.
52 Keller A., *Mainzer Kongressvortrage* 1957, 69:69.
53 Keys A., Henschel A. F., Taylor H. L., Mickelsen O., Brozek J., *Amer. J. Physiol* 1945, 144:5.
54 King C. G., 'Vitamin C' in *Handbook of Nutrition* publ. Amer. Med. Ass. Blakiston, N.Y., 1951.
55 ——*Nutr. Revs.* 1968, 26:33.
56 Kraybill H. F., Whitehair L. A., *Ann. Rev. Pharmacol.* 1967, 7:357.
57 Lawrence C., Klipstein F. A., *Ann. Int. Med.* 1967, 66:25.
58 Lowenstein L., Brunton L., Hseih Y-S., *Canad. Med. Ass. J.* 1966, 94:636.
59 ——Cantlie G., Ramos O., Brunton L., *Canad. Med. Ass. J.* 1966, 95:797.
60 Mackenzie C. G. in *Symposium on Nutrition* ed. R. M. Herriott, John Hopkins Press, Baltimore, 1953, p.136.
61 Majaj A. S., Dinning J. S., Azzam S. A., Darby W. J., *Amer. J. Clin. Nutr.* 1963, 12:374.
62 *Manual of Nutrition* publ. by Ministry Agric. Fish & Food, H.M.S.O. 1961.
63 Martin J. D., Davis R. E., *J. Obstet. Gynec. Brit. Comm.* 1964, 71:400.
64 Martin R. H., Marper T. A., Kelso W., *The Lancet* 1965, 1:670.
65 Marvin H. N., Audu I. S., *West African Med. J.* 1964, 13:3.
66 Masek J., *World Rev. Nutr. Dietet.* 1962, 3:177.
67 Mototh Y., Pinkas A., Sroka C., *Amer. J. Clin. Nutr.* 1965, 16:356.
68 *Medical Tribune* 1968, 3, no. 30, p.1.
69 Morgan T. B. Yudkin J., *Nature* 1957, 180:543.
70 Murphy E. W., Koons P. C., Page L., *J. Amer. Diet. Ass.* 1965, 55:372.
71 Najjar V A., Holt L. E., *J. Amer. Med. Ass.* 1943, 123:683.
72 *Nutrition Reviews* 1960, 18:182.
73 *Nutrition Reviews* 1962, 20:216.
74 Oldham H. G., Davis M. V., Roberts L. J., *J. Nutr.* 1944, 32:163.
75 Oski F. A., Barness L. A., *J. Amer. Med. Ass.* 1965, 193:47.
76 ——Barness L. A., *J. Pediatr.* 1967, 70:211.

77 *Recommended Dietary Allowances,* Nat. Res. Counc., Washington, D.C., 1953.
78 Richards M. G., *Brit. J. Nutr.* 1949, 3:132.
79 Schroeder H. A., *Amer. J. Clin. Nutr.* 1971, 24:562.
80 Sebrell W. H., Harris R. S., *The Vitamins,* Academic Press, N.Y. and London 1957.
81 Setyaadmadja A. T. S. H., Cheraskin E., Ringsdorf W. M., *J. Amer. Geriat. Soc.* 1965, 13:924.
82 Sinclair H. M., *Proc. Nutr. Soc.* (Lond.) 1958, 17:28.
83 Soskin P. A., Levine A. G., *Carbohydrate Metabolism,* Univ. of Chicago Press, Chicago 1952, p.19.
84 Streiff R. R., Little B., *J. Clin. Invest.* 1965, 44:1102.
85 Turchetti L. C., Cornbrink B., Krawitz S., Metz J., *Amer. J. Clin. Nutr.* 1966, 18:249.
86 Uhl E., *Amer. J. Clin. Nutr.* 1958, 6:146.
87 Varadi S., Elwis A., *The Lancet* 1964, 1:1162.
88 Venulet F., *Endokrinologie* 1953, 30:345.
89 Williams R. D., Mason H. L., Wilder R. M., Smith B. F., *Arch. Int. Med.* 1940, 66:785.
90 Willougby M. L. N., Jewel F. T., *Brit. Med. J.* 1966, 2:1568.
91 ——*Brit. J. Haematol.* 1967, 13:503.
92 Yefremov V. V., *Vopr. Pit.* 1958, 17:21.
93 Yudkin J., *Biochem. J.,* 1951, 48:608.
94 Ziporin Z. Z., Nunes W. T., Powell R. D., Waring P. P., Sauberlich H. E., *J. Nutr.* 1965, 85:297.

II In the elderly

1 Anderson I., Campbell A. E. R., Dunn A., Runciman J. B. M., *Scot. Med. J.* 1966, 11:429.
2 Andrews J., Brook M., *The Lancet* 1966, 1:1350.
3 —, — Allen M. A., *Geront. Clin.* 1966, 8:527.
4 Baker A. Z., *Geront. Clin.* 1962, 4:100.
5 Batata M., Spray G. H., Bolton F. E., Higgins G., Wollner L., *Brit. Med. J.* 1967, 2:667.
6 Beck J., Nordin B. E. C., *J. Path. Bact.* 1960, 80:391.
7 Bowers E. F., Kubik M. M., *Brit. J. Clin. Pract.* 1965, 19:141.
8 Brin M., Schwartzkopf D. A., Davies J., *J. Amer. Ger. Soc.* 1964, 12:493.
9 Brocklehurst J. C., Griffiths L L., Taylor G. F., Marks J., Scott J. L., Blackley J., *Geront. Clin.* 1968, 10:309.
10 Calder J. H., Curtis R. C., Fore H., *The Lancet* 1963, 1:556.
11 Collins D. H., in *Modern Trends in Diseases of Vertebral Column,* ed. R. Nassim, H. Jackson, p.101, Butterworth, London 1959.
12 Davison W., *Geront. Clin.* 1967, 9:393.
13 Dibble M. V., *J. Amer. Geriatics Soc.* 1967, 15:1031.
14 Drake R. M., Buechley R. W., Breslow L., Chope H. D., Address to West Amer. Publ. Health Assoc., Long Beach, Calif. 1957, cited by Morgan A. F., *Gerontologist* 1962, 2:77.
15 Exton Smith A. N., Stanton B. R., *Report on an Investigation into the Dietary of Elderly Women Living Alone,* King Edward's Hosp. Fund, London 1965.
16 Exton Smith A. N., Hodkinson H. M., Stanton B. R., *The Lancet* 1966, 2:999.

17 Forshaw J., Moorhouse E. H., Harwood L., *The Lancet* 1964, 1:1004.
18 Goran J., Green B., Mackay J., Walker W., *J. Coll. Gen. Pract.* 1965, 10:239
19 Gough K. R., Read A. E., McCarthy C. F., Waters A. H., *Quart J. Med.* 1963, 32:243.
20 ——Lloyd O. C., Wills M. R., *The Lancet* 1964, 2:1261.
21 Griffiths L. L., Brocklehurst J. C., Maclean R., Fry J., *Brit. Med. J.* 1966, 1:739.
22 —,—Scott D. L., Marks J., Blackley J., *Geront. Clin.* 1967, 9:1.
23 Hurdle A. D. F., Picton Williams T. C., *Brit. Med. J.* 1966, 2:202.
24 Kataria M. S., Rao D. B., Curtis R. C., *Geront. Clin.* 1965, 7:189.
25 Kirk J. E., Chieffi M., *Nutr.* 1949, 38:353.
26 Mills C. A., Cottingham E., Taylor E., *Arch. Biochem.* 1946, 9:221.
27 Milne J. S., Lonergan M. E., Williamson J., Moore F. M. L., *Brit. Med. J.* 1971, 4:383.
28 Morgan A. F., Gillm H. L., Williams R. I., *J. Nutr.* 1955, 55:413.
29 O'Sullivan D. J., Callaghan N., Ferrissa J. B., Finucane J. F., Hegarty M., *Irish J. Med. Sci.* 1968, 1:151.
30 Platt B. S., Eddy T. P., Pellett P. L., *Food in Hospitals* publ. Nuffield Provincial Hospitals Trust, London 1963.
31 Powell D. E. B., Thomas J. H., Mills P., *Geront. Clin.* 1968, 10:21.
32 Rafsky H. A., Newman B., *Geriatrics* 1947, 2:101.
33 Read A. E., Gough K. R., Pardoe J. L., Nicholas A., *Brit. Med. J.* 1965, 2:843.
34 Schulz F. H., Kirsch K., *Muenschen Med. Wochenschr* 1961, 103:1620.
35 Smith D. A., Harrison D., *Proc. Nutr. Soc., Lond.* 1968, 27:201.
36 Strachan R. W., Henderson J. G., *Quart. J. Med.* 1967, 36:189.
37 Taylor G. F., *The Lancet* 1966, 1:926.
38 Varadi S., Elwis A., *Brit. Med. J.* 1966, 2:410.
39 Wilson T. S., Weeks M. M., Mukherjee S. K., Murrell J. S., Andrews C. T., *Geron. Clin.* 1972, 14:17.
40 *World Medicine* 1968, 3:15.

Six

Mineral deficiencies

Changes in eating habits over the last hundred years have affected our mineral intake just as much as our vitamins. Deficiencies occur such as with iron and excesses occur as with sodium. Both can be harmful in different ways. In the world of trace element nutrition particularly, one is on new ground and possibilities are appearing of mineral imbalance. They are explored in this chapter. Two factors contribute to the mineral content of our food; (1) the way food is grown and on what soil, and (2) the processing and preparation of food. We are at the mercy of our environment in this respect as much as elsewhere.

Iron
Amongst women, low haemoglobin levels indicative of iron deficiency anemia, are common. Women lose blood in menstruation and do not partake of sufficient iron-rich foods to replace this loss. Estimates show that 15-25% of women have such anemia and as much as 35% have depleted body iron stores.

Scott and Pritchard[114] emphasize the frequency of low iron stores and low haemoglobin levels in America also. Amongst young women at college 66% possessed low to absent iron stores. Others in America[3, 56, 75, 92] report high prevalence of low haemoglobin levels in women rather than in men due to the blood loss that occurs with menstrual flow[29, 42, 59]. Elwood et al.[27] estimated the average loss of iron during menstruation at 13.5 mg per period in normal women necessitating an increased daily intake of iron in the diet to prevent depletion of body stores. That this amount of iron is not being presented in the diet or absorbed from the food is evident by the low marrow stores reported in young women.

103

Does this matter? Is there evidence of the female population suffering as a result of this depletion? Elwood[28] has painstakingly shown that many women have low haemoglobin levels and are *symptomless.* The condition is chronic and the physiology has adapted to it. He has also shown that symptoms of iron anaemia such as fatigue headache and breathlessness do not necessarily clear if the anaemia is cured by iron supplementation.[29, 122] Is it

TABLE 6.1
Surveys of prevalence of iron deficiency anaemia
in U.K.

Reference	Group studied	Criterion of anemia	% Anemic
Kilpatrick G. S., *Brit. Med. J.* 1961, 2:1736	145 women ages 15-24	< 12 G Hb/100 ml	28%
	25-34	,,	25%
	35-44	,,	24%
	45-54	,,	12%
	65-74	,,	21%
Kilpatrick G. S. et al., *Brit. Med. J.* 1961, 1:778.	200 women age 55-64	< 12 G Hb/100 ml	14%
Fry J., *Profiles of Disease.* Livingstone, Edin. 1966	2562 women over 10 yrs.	< 12 G Hb/100 ml	26.2%
Fielding J., et al., *The Lancet* 1965, 2:9	70 women	Estimation of Total Body Iron	35%
MacFarlane D. B. et al., *Brit. J. Haematol.* 1967, 13:794	500 women	< 12 G Hb/100 ml	11.6%
Elwood P. C., *Proc. Nutr. Soc.* 1968, 27:14	100 women	< 12 G Hb/100 ml	12%

therefore a significant morbid condition? These questions can only be answered by further research. Loh and Wilson[73] point out that vitamin C stores within the body are closely correlated with iron stores, and shortage of vitamin C in the diet can affect haemoglobin formation. Administration of iron can depress vitamin C levels in the blood, as the ascorbic acid is used in haemoglobin synthesis. Vitamin C supplementation is recommended at the same time as iron administration. It could well be that the anomalies uncovered by Elwood, the discrepancy between symptoms and haemoglobin level is simply due to the fact that these research workers are

104

looking at one parameter and not several. The body as a whole is being ignored.

Iron is found in the diet in meat, particularly liver, in cereals, eggs and vegetable. It is absorbed to greatest degree from meat,[57] to a smaller degree from cereals[30, 31] and eggs.[89] Vegetables are qualitatively a good source of mineral though not taken in abundance. However there is definite evidence that vitamin C[71] orange juice[10] and vegetables[70, 86] catalyse the absorption of iron from the jejunum and are important in this respect. Wholemeal bread has now definitely been shown to be a superior source of iron to refined white bread, enriched with iron.[11] The iron that is put into refined flour at the present time is virtually worthless due to lack of absorption.[30] Jacobs and Greenman[60] also highlight the very good iron absorption found in bran and All Bran. Maybe certain minerals in bran contribute to absorption efficiency.

Iron anemia should be taken seriously in the pregnant mother as risks are attached to anemia at this time,[12] complications of pregnancy being commoner in the anemic.[1, 7] Infants from anemic mothers are born anemic and suffer the effects of this handicap in the first year of life.[2] Nutritional education of young mothers is badly needed in this respect. Daily intake of iron is too low and the right foods are not being eaten.

Magnesium
Health food diets are rich in magnesium, for this mineral is found in abundance in nuts, wholegrain cereals, seafoods, meats, legumes and raw vegetables. Apart from the meat, most of these foods are advocated for consumption in health food journals. Wholegrain cereals contain magnesium for the refined flour loses magnesium in milling. Up to 80% of the mineral can be so lost. The situation is similar with rice. Cooking can also leach minerals from food and in the case of magnesium can effect a 33% - 40% loss. A similar situation is found with meat. A health food diet rich in the foods mentioned above could supply 500-600 mg of magnesium daily.

A 'normal' western diet or hospital diet supplies 200-260 mg of magnesium.[109, 112, 115] Duckworth and Warnock[26] in 1942 found intakes amongst the poorer classes as low as 200 mg. Amongst those better off, intakes rose to between 245 and 288 mg. Young college students in America at the present time have intakes that range from 200 to 400 mg of magnesium a day.[72] Irwin and Wiese[58] found six American students that averaged 319 mg intake and Leverton et al.[72] found that average intakes for three separate groups studied in America were 317, 263 and 244 mg. Diets rich in fat, sugar, meat and processed foods of one sort or another can be very low in magnesium content.[112] Whether high or low intakes of magnesium matter with regard to the health of man depends to an extent on the efficiency of the body's regulating mechanisms; the mechanisms that achieve homeostasis.

A low intake will not matter if (1) absorption from the intestine can be so increased as to compensate, and (2) renal excretion can be modified so as to conserve magnesium. Graham et al.[38] have shown that absorption is greatly increased on low dietary intake and Barnes, Cope and Harrison[4] have shown that renal conservation of magnesium on very low dietary intakes is extremely efficient. Conservation of magnesium has even been suggested as more efficient than that found operating for potassium or calcium.[74] It would seem that homeostasis can be achieved with a fair amount of ease.

Seelig[115] argues that deficiency as estimated by the presence of negative magnesium balance is commoner than realised in western countries and presents when daily magnesium intake falls below 420 mg. If Seelig is correct, and a lot of data has been collected by this research worker to support her thesis, most of us are deficient in magnesium. This is for the reason that normal intakes in Britain and America range from 200 mg to 300 mg, well below 420 mg. Seelig maintains that man is in negative balance below an intake of 420 mg. Negative balance requires the body to excrete more of a substance than is ingested. The body is thus losing a substance. But a loss of as small a quantity a day as 10 mg of magnesium would lead to total body depletion in 5 years and death would result. Obviously this does not happen to us and if one examines Seelig's data closer one observes that her figures for observed negative balance were taken over periods of only one to two weeks. Calcium balance is only achieved after months of duration, in some cases seven months. If magnesium is in any way similar to calcium, which is probable, a lot more time than two weeks should be allowed for the body to adapt to a certain intake and achieve balance. Malm[79] has shown how the body can adapt to low calcium intakes and Walker[121] has outlined native communities in Africa that exist on very low intakes of calcium. It is not unreasonable to expect the same situation with regard to magnesium. Schroeder[112] has discussed some of the above arguments in fuller detail in an article in the *Journal of Chronic Diseases*.

However if we are considering 'optimum health' it may not be enough for the body to achieve 'balance' with intake and output of nutrient whether it be vitamin or mineral. It has been shown that high intakes of vitamin C bring about certain positive effects within the body, as also vitamin B. Magnesium similarly may contribute advantages if fed in abundance. For instance it has been shown to lower cholesterol and retard the deposition of lipids in the aorta.[78, 120] The Bantu have high blood magnesium levels and low incidence of coronary disease.[6, 52] Magnesium has been shown to delay the formation of fibrin.[39] Hard water contains more magnesium than soft and hard water drinking consumption has now definitely been correlated with lower mortality from heart disease. [15, 16, 88, 90] Perhaps more important here are calcium/magnesium ratios or trace element content rather than solely the quantity of magnesium.[80]

Lack of magnesium has also been shown to play a possible role in the pathogenesis of renal stones, together however with many other factors. Bunce et al.[8] have shown that in rats a critical magnesium level exists above which renal stones cannot form. The magnesium in some way prevents stone formation. Others[33, 48, 65, 92] confirm the close relationship of magnesium levels and excretion to stone formation. Hammarsten[45, 46] many years ago showed that calcium oxalate deposition in the urine could be prevented by increasing intake of magnesium. Prien and others[37, 96] have confirmed this by administering magnesium along with vitamin B6 to sufferers from chronic renal lithiasis and reducing incidence remarkably.

It would seem therefore that magnesium is a valuable mineral, that has many uses within the body. A rich supply of this element would seem essential for full health. Refining of wholegrain cereals (rich in magnesium) and cooking of vegetables depletes the diet of magnesium. A modern diet low in magnesium foods (nuts, wholegrain cereals, seafoods, meats, legumes and raw vegetables) could prejudice health.

Calcium
Average adult intakes for calcium in this country range from 0.8

107

to 1.0 gm per day. Hegsted and others[50] in a recent symposium maintain that many poorer countries live on less calcium than this and do not suffer calcium deficiency as a result. Walker[50] gives examples of communities living on low calcium intakes and maintaining health, and where osteoporosis is prevalent in various countries, no relationship has been found to exist with rates of calcium intake.[36, 51]

In circumstances where volunteers, in prison, were put on low calcium intakes over a period of months, adaptation was found to occur in the body to decreased levels of calcium in the diet.[79] Adaptation took time to develop (in one case seven months) but almost always eventually occurred. The body adjusted itself and achieved balance even on intakes that were half the quantity of that ingested by western man nowadays. Hegsted et al. report similarly.[49] Efficiency of absorption has been shown to be higher in Ceylonese children than in American children.[91] The former eat less calcium. Macy[77] has shown the same phenomenon in a study with six boys. Three boys fed a standard diet absorbed 374 mg calcium a day. Another three boys fed a special high calcium diet for two months prior to the ordinary diet only absorbed 103 mg calcium per day. Their efficiency of absorption had been decreased by their previous luxury of calcium.

Sodium and potassium
It could be said that we eat too much sodium. Intakes of this mineral vary enormously according to taste and range between 5 and 20 gm a day amongst the population. Intakes of potassium on the other hand range between 2 and 5 gm. The ratio of sodium to potassium in the diet is therefore around 3:1 or 4:1. Meyer et al.[84] showed that for the rat, optimum growth took place at Na:K ratios of 1:2 and increasing the sodium intake to reach a ratio of 10:1, with potassium intake held steady, decreased the growth of rats. Ratios of sodium to potassium within this range have been recorded in Japan in areas of high mortality from cerebrovascular disease and hypertension.[99] Intakes of sodium though high are not at this level in this country.

In general, foods contain little sodium but more potassium, and he who is 'arguing from nature' could argue a case that it is more natural to take in potassium than sodium. In civilized countries we have reversed this balance and add salt to our food.

Salt, first used as a preservative, is now our common taste improver, and the more that food is cooked and processed the more the need for flavour to be added to it.

Food in its natural state however contains little sodium, and a lot of potassium. Sodium: potassium ratios in nuts for instance run from 1:200 to 1:800, and this on an analysis by weight. In fruits the ratio ranges from 1:200 to 1:4000 (found in bananas); in cereals 1:50 to 1:900. Vegetables have more sodium and the ratio therefore varies from 1:3 (spinach) to 1:40 (cabbage). Potatoes have a ratio of 1:600. Not till one considers eggs, milk and ordinary butter does the ratio drop to 1:3 or 1:1 (egg). Meat contains a fair amount of both minerals and ranges from 1:3 to 1:7. Food in its natural state therefore contains far more potassium than sodium. In effect this means that the body has to adapt to an unnaturally high sodium intake imposed upon it.

Excess sodium intake can be dealt with to an extent by the kidney and the hormonal regulating mechanisms of the body. The intake can also be balanced by increasing dietary potassium, but potassium containing foods, nuts, fruits, legumes and seeds are not eaten so regularly as the sodium rich foods in our society and this can lead to an imbalance.

Excess intake of salt has for some time in man been associated with hypertension. Dahl[23] marshals together much of the evidence for this relationship in a recent article. In man, much of the evidence is indirect.[18, 19, 64] It has been shown for instance that of 800 persons categorised as high, medium and low salt eaters, hypertension was present in the high salt group at 10%, in the medium group at 7% and the low group at 0%.[18] In Japan also, high salt intake has been correlated with increased incidence of hypertension.[99]

In animal experiments unequivocal hypertension has been produced now in rats by the feeding of sodium chloride and this condition in rats bears a remarkable similarity to the essential hypertension of man. In fact the clinical picture runs from slowly developing benign hypertension to early rapidly fatal malignant hypertension,[22, 83] just as in humans. Furthermore it is usually self sustained after salt removal.[20] Young animals are more susceptible than old and the longer the salt intake is maintained the more severe the hypertension induced.[24] Genetic factors[21] play a part and a big part in both rats and men and one has to remember this fact. Nevertheless there are dangers inherent in a high salt diet especially in infancy.

H. A. Guthrie[41] and L. K. Dahl[23] in the *American Journal of Nutrition* have drawn attention to the fact that tinned baby foods, commonly now fed to babies at the age of 2 months onwards, contain a greatly increased quantity of salt. So large is this addition and so widespread is the reliance placed upon these foods that both authors express great alarm at the hypertension that is liable to be induced in those genetically prone to this disease. Again it is stressed that in genetically susceptible rats it has been shown that even a transient high salt intake early in life will induce permanent, often fatal hypertension later.[24] Dahl estimates that a baby fed on tinned or jarred purée foods *can take in 8 times as much sodium as a baby on breast milk.* This could lead on evidence to certain hypertension if the child was genetically susceptible. Sodium is an unnecessary mineral to add to food. Furthermore it has been shown that a baby's palate does not require salt to titillate the appetite as might an adult's and if added as a preservative it is suggested that a more suitable compound be found immediately.

Trace elements

Trace element physiology is in its infancy. The field of research regarding these elements has only been gradually opened up in the last twenty years, though it promises interesting findings in the future. The field is unexplored and slightly mysterious, in its way, as the facts are often difficult of access. The quantities are minute but the data nevertheless extremely important. Trace elements should not be under-estimated for their effects upon man may prove to be far reaching. Indeed deficiencies in this field may be far more important to the health of man than those already discussed.

Four arguments will be initially presented to emphasize the contemporary importance of trace element study to the nutrition of man. It is thought by some that the study is *un*important for the reason that man is gregarious and his food orginates from a wide range of sources. It is therefore reasoned by some that he cannot suffer deficiency of trace elements as a result of food ingestion. Four points are put forward here to counter this point of view.

(1) Geographically, variations occur in amount of trace elements found in the soil. Deficiences of certain elements occur in certain areas and predispose to disease. Examples of this are iodine

110

deficiency leading to goitre, fluoride deficiency leading to dental caries,[25, 81] and osteoporosis,[5] molybdenum deficiency leading to dental caries,[9] molybdenum deficiency leading to oesophageal cancer[47] and copper deficiency possibly playing a role in increased cancer incidence.[47] All these deficiencies relate to soil deficiencies in specific geographical areas. Disease prevalence varies with the soil type.

(2) The food of man is becoming divorced from the soil. Refining of flour removes minerals from flour, and any form of heating and preparing in water or steam leaches out minerals from food. Refined sugar, a substance eaten in quantity contains virtually no minerals at all. All this might not matter if man ate a balanced and varied diet. Evidence presented in this book suggests that a sizeable proportion of the population do not. If the diet is in any way prejudiced against the inclusion of fruit, and vegetables, a certain degree of mineral and trace element deficiency could be expected. Plant foods in general are a rich source of minerals; nuts, legumes and wholegrain cereals contributing.

(3) The industrial environment of modern times has introduced other elements, besides those that are essential, into man's body. Examples of such substances include lead, tin, cadmium, barium, germanium, titanium, arsenic and mercury. These may interfere with normal mineral metabolism, and cause deficiency and disease.

(4) Modern agricultural practices involve the application of mineral fertilisers to the soil. This can upset trace element balance within the soil and alter uptake by plants and cereals. Liming can inhibit the release and uptake of cobalt, nickel, manganese and zinc from the soil.[105] The application of superphosphate can lead to copper deficiency[113] and suppress the uptake of niobium and vanadium[106] while the over application of phosphate can lead to zinc deficiency.[95] Potash application can induce boron soil deficiency.[113] But perhaps the greatest problem that attaches to modern agricultural practices, and particularly in America, relates to the amount of mineral taken out of soil compared to that put back into soil. It is obviously impossible to regulate by such means the exact replacement of trace minerals. Organic manures have the advantage of containing an abundance of such minerals within them but such manuring is difficult and expensive to accomplish under modern management conditions. There is therefore risk of soil

mineral depletion in many cases. Soil deficiencies of zinc, copper, magnesium and manganese are becoming commoner in agricultural practice. Other examples are likely to occur. Such deficiencies could predispose to human deficiency if widespread. There is however a great lack of knowledge concerning these matters at the present time.

Dr. H. A. Schroeder in America has done perhaps most work regarding trace element requirement in the human and regards eleven trace elements, so far, as essential to man. They are iron, chromium, manganese, cobalt, zinc, selenium, molybdenum, iodine, copper, vanadium and nickel.[105] Altogether 29 trace metals are found in man which leads one to suppose that 18 of these are either contaminants or undiscovered biological agents. No doubt some of them will be found to fall into the second category as time proceeds.

Trace elements by their very name exist in minute quantities in the environment. They can sometimes constitute less than 0.01% of the environmental medium. The sense of ridicule that originally attached to this fact and their appearance in such minute quantities has fortunately passed, for scientific experiment has now revealed the potency of such substances. It is now common knowledge, for instance, that fluoride can act at concentrations of 1 part per million to affect dental caries. Many trace elements act as catalysts to enzymatic reactions in human physiology though their role in many respects is ill understood. Some, such as vanadium are inhibitory in action, others such as copper excitatory. Most elements work at highest efficiency in an optimum environment which is dependent upon exact concentrations of other mineral constituents. This dependency leads one to consider these trace elements more in terms of an *integrated team* than as individual catalysts. Present knowledge of the exact working of this team is even less than the knowledge acquired concerning the individual components and one can only hope that more will be found out regarding them in the future.

Zinc

Foods that are rich in zinc are seafoods, meats, wholegrains, dairy produce, legumes and nuts.[109] Vegetables are a relatively poor source. Adequate amounts of zinc are supposed to be present in western diets. A diet poor in such foods as eggs, wholegrain

112

cereals, liver, beans and peas would be low in zinc, but on the whole most of us eat some of these foods.

In poverty areas of the Middle East, frank zinc deficiency has been diagnosed[94, 98] but not in western countries. Here we have to look more for subclinical symptomatology regarding the pathogenesis of chronic disease. Low blood levels of zinc however have been found in a number of diseases such as diabetes, chronic tuberculosis, chronic infections and azotemia. Women who are pregnant or taking oral contraceptives have lower blood zinc levels.[43]

Zinc has been shown to play a part in spermatogenesis, and it is known to concentrate in the prostate of the male. Zinc has also been shown to concentrate in hair, which tissue becomes deficient in the mineral following dietary depression. The mineral has also been shown to aid skeletal growth and has been shown to be a constituent of many essential enzymes in the human body including alkaline phosphatases and certain dehydrogenases.[69] Adequate zinc is as important to the body's physiology as adequate iron. Therapeutically zinc has aided wound healing,[93] halving time of wound closure, and has improved exercise tolerance in the claudicated lower limb.[118] The ratio of zinc: cadmium, zinc: copper and zinc: calcium within the human body may bear importantly upon health.

High calcium uptake depresses zinc uptake and conversely a high zinc intake depresses calcium uptake. The relationship also exists between copper and zinc. It has been shown to hold in pigs.[53] A high zinc intake can depress copper uptake, while presence of copper can assist for its part in preventing zinc deficiency.[53] That these relationships are more than just academic is shown by the research into the epidemiology of gastric cancer, initiated by Stocks in North Wales.[117] Stocks noted that soil from the gardens of patients who had died from cancer of the stomach had high zinc levels and low copper content. Zinc can provoke copper deficiency in the soil. The copper deficiency was postulated as a factor in the epidemiology of this cancer. The theory could not obviously hold unless one ate vegetables grown from one's own garden. These patients were shown to be rural in habits and to so derive their vegetables.

However the local water supply can give as much variation in mineral content as the soil, and also present as an epidemiological factor in cancer. Hargreaves,[47] inspired by the work of

Stocks, analysed the zinc and copper concentrations in the water supply of various towns in Cornwall.

Different zinc/copper ratios correlated with different rates for cancer mortality and correlated also with prevalence figures for multiple sclerosis. Suggestions were made that the zinc and copper affected aetiology of these diseases.

Throughout the soils of America, the situation is one of Zinc deficiency.[95] High levels of crop production, the presence of alkaline soils, leached acidic soils, superphosphate fertilization, and the lack of organic manures have all contributed to a deficiency that is becoming as widespread in some quarters as nitrogen deficiency. Some 32 states throughout America report this deficiency and Australia, New Zealand, Brazil and Western Europe have all recently noted increases in zinc deficiency in soils. Reasons given for this include the fact that mechanisation brings less organic manuring. Zinc taken out of the soil is not replaced. Fewer cattle are fed from farm crops. More and more farms have no livestock at all. Older forms of phosphate manure were 'impure' and the manures contained trace elements. Phosphate fertiliser contemporarily is a purified product. Zinc and other trace metals *are not replaced to the same extent as previously.* Intensive arable cropping can deplete the soil of these essential elements. The effects upon human health of new methods of agriculture in this respect have not been studied. They are for the most part a mystery. If human hypertensives have a high cadmium/low zinc content in their tissues, as is shown further on, is this possibly the result of environmental changes· that have been brought about by newer methods of farming? The question cannot be answered till more work is done upon it, but opens up possibilities.

Cadmium and zinc

Cadmium is not an essential trace element. On the contrary it is toxic to animal and man on accumulation. When fed to rats it produces hypertension, increases mortality and shortens the life span.[104] If injected into dogs, retention of sodium occurs from interference with the function of the proximal convoluted tubule. This may be the route by which hypertension is caused in man and animal. Human hypertensives have been found to excrete far more cadmium than controls and those dying from hypertension had increased cadmium content of their tissues or an increase in the cadmium/zinc ratio.[104] Rats in small doses developed hypertension which reverted to normal on withdrawing the cadmium from their diet.

Schroeder argues that our intake of this trace element is harmfully high in the western world and arises from modern environmental hazards. Refining bread, flour or rice in the case of cadmium increases the concentration of the mineral rather than decreasing it, for cadmium is contained in the starchy endosperm. Cadmium/zinc ratios in whole wheat flour are 1/65 and in refined flour 1/26. Schroeder[109] holds that these ratios of mineral intake are important as far as the toxicology of the element is concerned as the imbalance affects concentrations within the body. The processing of foods is similarly a mechanism that raises cadmium concentrations and processed tomatoes, milk and cereal have been shown to have a significantly higher concentration of cadmium than the natural product.[100] Seafoods are a natural food high in cadmium. Coffee and tea contain a fair amount. The Japanese eat both seafoods and refined rice. They also have an incidence of hypertension much higher than the Americans. Tissue levels of cadmium in post mortem tissues were also higher in the Japanese than the Americans.[100] The mineral accumulates in the kidney. These and other facts have led Schroeder to consider cadmium as a toxic nutritional trace element and an agent in the genesis of hypertension.

An important point, however, admitted by these workers themselves, that argues against this thesis is the fact that labourers working in cadmium dust do not develop hypertension.[104] Is the ratio of cadmium to other minerals ingested perhaps different here in some respect? Further research will no doubt elucidate this particular point, but meanwhile some suspicion is cast upon the processing of food and the mineral and trace element changes that occur as a result. The story is the same for chromium.

Chromium
Chromium is not found abundantly in human foods. It is of far greater abundance in wild forage foods.[101] The refining of flour lowers chromium levels in bread and the consumption of sugar increases the need for the mineral, for sucrose mobilises chromium from the tissues and leads to excretion of the mineral.[111] Heating of

food to high levels can also destroy chromium content. With refined flour, sugar and cooked food which are so basic to modern dietary habits, contributing to chromium deficiency it is hardly surprising that low tissue levels are found in adult man. Whether this matters is another question. It could be that an important deficiency here arises that affects the pathogenesis of both heart disease and diabetes.

Chromium appears to be a trace element essential for optimal growth and longevity in rats and the prevention of spontaneous aortic plaques in rats.[110] Chromium deficiency also produces an increase in blood lipids and a disturbance of glucose tolerance.[103] Administration of chromium to infants with kwashiorkor who possessed diabetic glucose tolerance tests, cured the diabetic tendency in some cases.[55, 111] Its use has therefore been suggested in the treatment of diabetes in man.[54]

Physiologically chromium increases cholesterol and fatty acid synthesis, and assists insulin in the deposition of fat within the body.[101] It has been shown to be present at birth in the new born baby but only present at very low levels in later years. It appears therefore to disappear from body tissues as age advances. Schroeder estimates this is due to dietary deficiency rather than decreased need. In tissues of peoples from countries showing low incidence of heart disease, levels of chromium are high into adult age. By contrast, 17.6% of American tissues are *quite deficient in chromium.* This could be an important deficiency.

Copper

This element is ubiquitous, and present in most foods. High intakes are therefore simple to achieve, for seafoods, meat, eggs, nuts, fruit, cereals contain a lot of the mineral. Copper is a catalyst in many oxidative processes, affecting coenzyme A[40] and many lipid enzyme systems[113] that involve phospholipid metabolism. Malnourished infants given high calorie food intake may develop a copper deficiency by increased growth demands.[13] Mention has been made previously of certain findings as regards zinc/copper ratios in soil and the relationship to gastric cancer. This element may play a protective role against cancer. A deficiency could present in certain geographical locations, which would affect the pathogenesis of chronic disease. On the whole deficiency is unlikely.[108]

116

Molybdenum

Molybdenum is an essential trace element to man and in two notable pieces of epidemiological detection has been shown to play a preventive role in medicine. This has involved dental caries in one instance and the prevention of oesophageal cancer in another.

Trace elements have been known to affect incidence of dental caries for some years. It is perhaps due to the accessibility of the human tooth for purposes of study that so many factors have been found to influence progress of caries in man. It is not unreasonable to expect that other diseases in man might similarly be linked to trace element nutriture in time to come. Vanadium,[37] boron,[67] lithium[116] strontium and fluorine[81] are all trace elements that affect tooth nutrition.

Molybdenum can be added to this list as the result of some interesting detection work that was carried out epidemiologically in New Zealand.[61, 76] Two towns figured in this survey, one called Napier and the other called Hastings. Napier showed a lower incidence of dental caries in children than Hastings and was built on a marine soil that had a different trace mineral content to Hastings. Napier's soil contained more molybdenum, aluminium and titanium. Hastings soil on the other hand contained more manganese, copper, barium and strontium. The most significant difference was in molybdenum content. Napier vegetables contained ten times as much of this mineral as those from Hastings. The teeth of Napier children also contained more of this element.

Some rather neatly performed animal experiments confirmed the role that molybdenum was playing in preventing dental caries. The vegetables grown from the two locations were ashed and the ash was fed to rats. Caries incidence in the rats again varied, being less on Napier ash than Hastings. In place of Napier ash, molybdenum was then fed the rats and caries prevented to an almost identical degree.

Molybdenum also appears to affect the incidence of oesophageal cancer by its presence in the soil.[68] In South Africa for instance over ten years a rise in incidence of this cancer has occurred. Dr. Burrell in surveying the gardens of those who had died from oesophageal cancer, rather as Stocks had done in North Wales for gastric cancer, found that signs of molybdenum deficiency were present in the gardens of these patients, following vegetable and soil analysis. The patients were all rural patients who had sub-

117

sisted on garden produce over some period. Control gardens had normal molybdenum levels. The molybdenum deficient plants were however susceptible to fungal attack and a strong possibility presented itself that the breakdown products of the disease — nitrosamines — caused the cancer as much as the molybdenum deficiency.[9]

Refining and processing destroys trace elements
Refining of flour and processing procedures such as canning take away minerals and trace elements from the food as well as vitamins. Schroeder[107] shows in a summary of this problem that deficiencies are occurring in the American diet of zinc, manganese and chromium. Comparing canned foods to the raw product, canned spinach lost 81.7% of the manganese, 70.6% of the cobalt, 40% of the zinc. Zinc losses amounted to 60% in canned beans and 83.3% in canned tomatoes. White bread as compared with whole wheat bread was lower in magnesium by 40%, in chromium by 71.4%, in cobalt by 69.4%, in copper by 69.8%, and in zinc by 77.4%. When a food is divided into its component parts by refinement or extraction, trace metals are in danger of being lost. Refined sugar has virtually no trace minerals left in it. Marked loss of trace metals occurs when rice is polished.

Schroeder[107] *in analysing diets commonly eaten in America found foods low in manganese, zinc, copper, selenium, molybdenum and chromium.* He emphasises the need to investigate these deficiencies more closely. Trace minerals are found abundantly in such foods as raw vegetable, whole grains, seafoods, nuts, and some meats.

Finale
Man's absolute dependence upon any one trace element is always hard to prove for reasons already mentioned. Simple deficiency in man is unethical to produce. Relative deficiency has to be inferred from various biological data. In respect of some of the lesser known elements certain actions within human metabolism have been shown to exist. Manganese interacts with choline and is responsible for a lipotropic action.[14] It is excreted in the bile and is responsible for such actions within the body as oxidation to carbon dioxide within the citric acid cycle.[85] Vanadium has an anti-atherosclerotic action[113] and decreases plasma lipid and cholesterol levels by an

118

inhibiting action upon cholesterol synthesis.[17] Vanadium may also play a vital role in the mineralization of teeth and bones.[119] Nickel is probably concerned with pigmentation in man and biology of the epithelium.[102] It behaves like a trace element in that it is ubiquitous in nature, present in both plants and mammals, present at human birth, has a low molecular weight and is relatively non-toxic.[102] Selenium forms lipid antioxidants that have a hundred times the activity of alpha tocopherol (vitamin E), and function in vivo like alpha tocopherol.[44] It is therefore conceivable that selenium spares vitamin E in body metabolism and plays an important role in fat metabolism.

Most trace elements are found widespread over a range of foods and as in the case of copper it is difficult to sustain a deficiency of any one of them if a varied balanced diet is taken. However the foods richest in trace elements, the wholegrains, seafoods, legumes, nuts, fruits and vegetables are not eaten to the extent that they might be in certain sectors of the population. *Trace elements are refined out of cereals to an extent, and are frequently lost in processing and cooking of food. There thus exists a possibility that deficiency could present on a monotonous mediocre or poorly chosen diet.* Schroeder considers such deficiency might arise in the case of zinc, chromium and possibly other under-studied elements such as manganese. At the moment the whole field lacks investigation and needs much research. Two factors in our modern environment could contribute to a change in trace element availability. The one concerns modern agricultural practices associated with high output production and selected mineral fertilisation, that can alter trace element content of soils. The second concerns the processing of food which involves possible contamination *and* depletion of trace element content. Food habits are at the moment changing rapidly. Our mineral nutrition could be changing with them, and for the worse.

To summarise, analyses of diets recently carried out in America found foods low in Manganese, Zinc, Copper, Selenium, Molybdenum and Chromium. Magnesium is lost to a great extent in cereals in the refining process though as with Calcium the body is efficient in retaining and conserving Magnesium. Iron deficiency is the commonest of all deficiencies and the situation can be shown to be serious in the case of young women who show high incidence of marrow depletion. The type of food we eat today has lowered the intake of certain minerals, but the total effect of this upon our health requires to be assessed. The body can adjust to low intakes of a mineral but one must ask, how low, at what expense and is the adjustment detrimental to full health. These questions are largely unanswered.

REFERENCES TO CHAPTER 6

1 Afonina L. G., *A Kuserstsvo Ginekol* 1965, No. 4.66 (*Nut. Abst. Rev.* 1966, 36:3250).
2 ——*Pediatrija* 1965, 44:59 (*Nut. Abst. Rev.* 1965, 35:6583).
3 Allaire B. I., Campagna A., *Obstet. gynec.* 1961, 17:605.
4 Barnes B. A., Cope O., Harrison T., *J. Clin Invest.* 1958, 37:430.
5 Bernstein D. S., Sadowsky N., Hegsted D. M., Guri C. D., Stare F. J., *J. Amer. Med. Ass.* 1966, 198:499.
6 Bersohn I., Oelofse P. J., *The Lancet* 1957, 1:1020.
7 Black D. A. K., Milne M. D., *Clin. Sci.* 1952, 11:397.
8 Bunce G. E., Sauberlich H. E., Oba T. S., *J. Nutr.* 1965, 86:406.
9 Burrell R. J. W., Roach W. A., Shadwell A., *J. Nat. Cancer Inst.* 1966, 36:201.
10 Callender S T., Warner G. T., *Amer. J. Clin. Nutr.* 1968, 21:1170.
11 ——Warner G. T., *The Lancet* 1970, 1:546.
12 Chanarin I., Rothman D., Berry V., *Brit. Med. J.* 1965, 1:485.
13 Cordano A., Baertl J. M., Graham G. G., *Pediatr.* 1964, 34:324.
14 Cotzias G. C., *Physiol. Rev.* 1958, 38:503.
15 Crawford M. D., Gardner M. J., Morris J. N., *The Lancet* 1968, 1:827.
16 Crawford T., Crawford M. D., *The Lancet* 1967, 1:229.
17 Curran G. L., Azarnoff D. L., Bolinger R. E., *J. Clin. Invest.* 1959, 38:1251.
18 Dahl L. K., Love R. A., *Arch. Int. Med.* 1954, 94:525.
19 ——in *Essential Hypertension. An International Symposium*, ed. P. T. Cottier, K. D. Bock., publ. Springer, Heidelberg 1960, p.3.
20 ——*J. Expl. Med.* 1961, 114:231.
21 ——Heine M. A., Tassinari L., *J. Expl. Med.* 1962, 115:1173.
22 —— Schackow E., *Can. Med. Ass. J.* 1964, 90:155.
23 ——*Amer. J. Clin. Nutr.* 1968, 21:787.
24 ——Knudsen K. D., Heine M. A., Leitl G. J., *Circulation Res.* 1968, 22:11.
25 Dean H. T., Arnold F. A., Elvove E., *Publ. Health Rep.* 1942, 66:1389.
26 Duckworth J., Warnock G. M., *Nutr. Abst. Rev.* 1942, 12:167.
27 Elwood P. C., Rees G., Thomas J. D. R., *Brit. J. Prev. Soc. Med.* 1968, 22:127.
28 ——*Brit. Med. J.* 1967, 4:714.
29 ——*Proc. Nutr. Soc.* 1968, 27:14.
30 ——*Iron in Flour* Reports on Public Health and Medical Subjects No. 117 H.M.S.O. 1968.
31 ——Newton D., Eakins J. D., Brown D. A., *Amer. J. Clin. Nutr.* 1968, 21:1162.
32 Epstein F. H., *Amer. J. Med.* 1968, 45:700.

33 Evans R. H., Forbes M. A., Sutton R. A. L., Watson L., *The Lancet* 1967, 2:958.
34 Fielding J., O'Shaughnessy M. C., Brunstrom G. M., *The Lancet* 1965, 2:9.
35 Fry J., *Profiles of Disease*, Livingstone, Edinburgh, London 1966, p.92.
36 Garn S. M., Rohmann C. G., Wagner B., *Fed. Proc.* 1967, 26:1729.
37 Gershoff S. N., Prien E. L., *Amer. J. Clin. Nutr.* 1967, 20:393.
38 Graham L. A., Caesar J. J., Burgen A. S. V., *Metabolism* 1960, 9:646.
39 Greville G. D., Lehmann H., *J. Physiol.* 1944 103:175.
40 Gubler C. J., *J. Amer. Med. Ass.* 1956, 161:530.
41 Guthrie H. A., *Amer. J. Clin. Nutr.* 1968, 21:863.
42 Hallberg L., Hogdahl A. M., Nillsson L., Rybo G., *Acta Obstet. Gynec. Scand.* 1966, 45:320.
43 Halsted J. A., Smith J. C., *The Lancet* 1970, 1:322.
44 Hamilton J. W., Tappel A. L., *J. Nutr.* 1963, 79:493.
45 Hammarsten G., *Compt. Rend. Trav. Lab.* Carlsberg 1929, 17:1.
46 ——in *Etiologic Factors in Renal Lithiasis* ed. A. J. Butt, Charles C. Thomas, Springfield, Ill. 1956.
47 Hargreaves E. R., In *Symposium of Health in a Changing Environment* J. Coll. Gen. Pract. 1966 suppl. 1.12, p.24.
48 Heaton F. W., Anderson C. K., *Clin. Sci.* 1965, 28:99.
49 Hegsted D. M., Moscosco I., Collazos C., *J. Nutr.* 1952, 46:181.
50 ——*J. Amer. Med. Ass.* 1963, 185:588.
51 ——*Fed. Proc.* 1967, 26:1747.
52 Higginson J., Pepler W. J., *J. Clin. Invest.* 1954, 33:1366.
53 Hoekstra W. G., *Fed. Proc.* 1964, 23:1068.
54 Hopkins L. L., Majaj A. S., *Fed. Proc.* 1966, 25:303.
55 ——Ransome Kuti O., Majaj A. S., *Amer. J. Clin. Nutr.* 1968, 21:203.
56 Hunter C. A., *Surg. Gynec. Obstet.* 1960, 110:210.
57 Hussain R., Walker R. B., Layrisse M., Clark P., Finch C. A., *Amer. J. Clin. Nutr.* 1965, 16:464.
58 Irwin M. I., Wiese H. F., *J. Nutr.* 1961, 74:217.
59 Jacobs A., Butler E. B., *The Lancet* 1965, 2:407.
60 ——Greenman D. A., *Brit. Med. J.* 1969, 1:673.
61 Jenkins G. N., *Brit. Dent. J.* 1967, 122:435.
62 Kilpatrick G. S., *Brit. Med. J.* 1961, 2:1736.
63 ——Hardisty R. M., *Brit. Med. J.* 1961, 1:78.
64 Knudsen K. D., Dahl L. K., *Postgrad. Med.* 1966, 42:148.
65 Ko K. W., Fellers F. X., Craig J. M., *Lab. Invest.* 1962, 11:294.
66 Kohler F. P., Uhle C. A. W., *J. Urol.* 1966, 96:812.
67 Kruger B. J., *Aust. Dent. J.* 1958, 3:236.
68 *The Lancet* 1966, 1:1145.
69 *The Lancet* 1968, 2:268.
70 Layrisse M., Martinez-Torres C., Roche M., *Amer. J. Clin. Nutr.* 1968, 21:1175.
71 Lee P. C., Ledwich J. R., Smith D. C., *Can. Med. Ass. J.* 1967, 97:181,
72 Leverton R. M., Leichsenring J. M., Linkswiler H., Meyer F., *J. Nutr.* 1961, 74:33.
73 Loh H. S., Wilson C. W. M. *The Lancet* 1971, 2:768.
74 Lowe K. G., *Clin. Sci.* 1953, 12:57.
75 Lund C. J., *Amer. J. Obstet. Gynec.* 1951, 62:947.
76 Ludwig T. G., Cadell P. B., Malthus R. S., *Int. Dent. J.* 1964, 14:433.
77 Macy I. G., *Nutrition and Chemical Growth in Childhood*, vol. 1

The food and health of western man

Evaluation, Charles C. Thomas, Springfield, Ill. 1942.
78 Malkiel-Shapiro B., Bersohn I., Terner P. E., *Med. Proc.* 1956, 2:455.
79 Malm O. J., *Scan J., Clin. Lab. Invest.* 1958, 10: supp. 36.
80 Marier J., Rose D., *Brit Med. J.* 1963, 2:686.
81 McClure F. J., Likins R. C., *J. Dent. Res.* 1951, 30:172.
82 McFarlane D. B., Pinkerton P. H., Dagg J. H., Goldberg A., *Brt. J. Haematol* 1967, 13:794.
83 Meneely G. R., Tucker R. G., Darby W. J., Auerbach S. H., *J. Exptl. Med.* 1953, 98:71.
84 Meyer J. H., Grunert R. R., Zepplin M. T., Grummer R. H., Bohstedt G., Phillips R. H., *Amer. J. Physiol.* 1950, 162:182.
85 Monty K. J., McElroy N. D., in *Food the Yearbook of Agriculture* ed. A. Stefferud. Govt. printing office, Washington D.C. 1959.
86 Moore C. V., *Amer. J. Clin. Nutr.* 1955, 3:3.
87 Morgan R. H., M.D. thesis Cambridge Univ. 1965.
88 Morris J., Crawford M.D., Heady J. A., *The Lancet* 1961, 1:860.
89 Narula K. K., Wadsworth G. R., *Proc. Nutr. Soc.* 1968, 27:No. 1. 13A.
90 Neal J. B., Neal M., *Arch. Path.* 1962, 73:58.
91 Nicholls L., Nimalasuriya A., *J. Nutr.* 1939, 18:563
92 Oreopoulos D. G., Soyannwo M.A.O., McGeown M.G., *The Lancet* 1968, 2:420.
93 Pories W. J., Heazel J. H., Rob C. G., Strain W. H., *The Lancet* 1967, 1:121.
94 Prasad A. S., Miale A., Farid J., Sanstead H. H., Schulert A. R., Darby W. J., *Arch. Int. Med.* 1963, 111:407.
95 ——*Zinc Metabolism* Charles C. Thomas, Springfield, Ill. 1966.
96 Prien E. L., *J. Amer. Med. Ass.* 1965 192:177 (*J. Nutr.* 1965, 86:406).
97 Pritchard J. A., Hunt C. F., *Surg. gynec. obst.* 1958, 106:516.
98 Sanstead H. H., Shukry A. S., Prasad A. S., Gabr. M. K., Mokhtar A. N., Darby W. J., *Amer. J. Clin. Nutr.* 1965, 17:15.
99 Sasaki N., *Japan Heart J.,* 1962, 3:313.
100 Schroeder H. A., Balassa J. J., *J. Chron. Dis.* 1961, 14:236.
101 ——*J. Chron. Dis.* 1962, 15:941.
102 ——Balassa J. J., Tipton I. H., *J. Chron. Dis.* 1962, 15:51.
103 ——Vinton W. H., Balassa J. J., *J. Nutr.* 1963, 80:48.
104 ——*J. Chron. Dis.* 1965, 18:647.
105 ——*J. Chron. Dis.* 1965, 18:217.
106 ——*J. Chron. Dis.* 1965, 18:229.
107 ——*Amer. J. Clin. Nutr.* 1971, 24:562.
108 ——Nason A. P., Tipton I. H., *J. Chron. Dis.* 1966, 19:1007.
109 ——Nason A. P., Tipton I. H., Balassa J. J., *J. Chron. Dis.* 1967, 20:179.
110 ——*Circulation* 1967, 35:570.
111 ——*Amer. J. Clin. Nutr.* 1968, 21:230.
112 ——Nason A. P., Tipton I. H., *J. Chron. Dis.* 1969, 21:815.
113 Schutte K. H., *The Biology of the Trace Elements,* Crosby Lockwood, London 1964.
114 Scott D. E., Pritchard J. A., *J. Amer. Med. Ass.* 1967, 199:897.
115 Seelig M. S., *Amer. J. Clin. Nutr.* 1964, 14:342.
116 Shaw J. H., Griffiths D., *Arch oral. Biol.* 1961, 5:301.
117 Stocks P., Davies R. E., *Brit. J. Cancer* 1964, 18:14.
118 Strain H., Pories W. H., *J. Amer. Med. Ass.* 201:No. 6. p.43.
119 Underwood E. J., *Trace Elements in Human and Animal Nutrition,*

2nd ed. N.Y. Academic Press 1962.
120 Vitale J. J., White P. L., Nakawara M., Zamchek N., *J. Exp. Med.* 1957, 106:757.
121 Walker A. R. P., Fox F. W., Irving J. T., *Biochem J.* 1948, 42:453.
122 Wood M. M., Elwood P. C., *Brit. J. Prev. Soc. Med.* 1966, 20:117.

Seven

Soil, food and health

It should be a statement of the obvious to say that soil health and human health are closely linked, or that the nutrition of the soil affects the nutrition of man. But it is not. In this technological age, we divorce ourselves from the soil and lose our links with Mother Earth. Food is 'grown in factories', wrapped and processed by industry, and 'has nothing to do' with the earth, and what is in the earth. Only when vegetables are grown in our own back garden do we associate health of soil with health of plant and *possibly* then our own health. The relationship otherwise does not impress itself upon our attention and understanding. We are indeed in this day and age divorced from the soil, and as a consequence have little understanding of the relationship that soil health bears to human health.

Soil
Soil is a complex dynamic living entity. The soil is not solid. It is actually composed of billions of grains of soil particles ranging from 1/2000 of an inch to 1/12 of an inch in diameter. Each of these tiny soil particles is covered with a tight-fitting film of oxides, water and organic matter. This provides the habitation for the teeming soil life. The surface area of these particles is staggering. One ounce of soil can have surfaces adding up to 250,000 square feet—about six acres! Within the top few inches of healthy soil are found bacteria, fungi, moulds, yeasts, protozoa, algae, worms, insects and other minute organisms. The bacteria alone may number up to 3 or 4 billion in a single gram of soil. This hive of activity serves the needs of the plant growing in such soil. The health of this community determines the health of the

124

plant, and ultimately the health of man. It is the aim of this chapter to point to certain evidence which emphasises the links which exist between soil, plant and man, and which bind man in his physiology and health to the soil on which he stands. These links are subtle and evidence for them is slow to accumulate. The right experiments are still waiting to be done, and the data to be collected.

Manurial treatment and plant health
(1) *Trace elements*
The soil is a complex of inorganic and organic mineral complexes. To add mineral fertiliser to the soil of whatever quality will tend to upset this delicate balance. An undue emphasis on N, P, and K (nitrate, phosphate and potash fertilisers) as additives will inevitably depress naturally occurring forms of mineral supply, and lock up availability of trace elements. The availability of trace elements has been shown to be less in certain soils farmed intensively and new trace deficiencies seem always to be appearing. It is probable that N, P, and K can depress natural mineral availability by simple laws of mass action and ionic diffusion but also by adversely affecting the bacterial population of the soil. Webley[4] has shown that certain bacteria of the root zone release soluble phosphates from the soil and he has also shown that silica, aluminium, calcium, manganese and calcium are all solubilised by the action of the bacteria from their insoluble fractions within the soil.[10]

Brown and Albrecht[5] have detailed how iron, manganese, copper and boron availability levels have all been depressed in soils artificially fertilised, and the works of Voisin[30, 31] go into considerable detail over trace element depression following mineral fertilisation. Voisin shows how copper levels can be depressed by nitrogen fertilisation, zinc by phosphoric acid, how magnesium, calcium and sodium are affected by potash application, manganese by chalk, and so on. He also shows how manganese availability in the soil can affect vitamin C content of Brussels sprouts, and calcium and potash fertilisation the carotene content of beet leaves, how nitrogenous fertilisation can affect riboflavin levels in spinach, and how excess potassium fertilisation can lower the blood levels of magnesium in cows fed on grass subject to such a regime.

Others have confirmed how the trace element nutrition of plant can affect nutritional quality of produce.[13] Manganese, boron and

125

iron increase sugar and ascorbic acid content of tomatoes.[16, 28] Trace element balance within the soil affects vitamin content of carrots, cabbage, clover, beans and maize.[12, 15] Greenhouse tomatoes top dressed with boron, copper, magnesium and manganese increased their ascorbic acid content.[16] Amino acid composition of fruit is affected by trace element deficiency.[17] That these elements work at incredibly small concentrations is shown by the research of Ahmed and Jones.[1] Working with cobalt, Ahmed and Jones showed that concentrations of one part in ten thousand million of cobalt increased the dry weight of soya bean by 69%! All this evidence confirms the place of trace elements in crop nutrition. If N.P. and K are liable to affect this balance detrimentally, lock up or change the balance of microelements within the soil, then nutritional quality of produce almost certainly will be affected. Prasad[19] maintains that zinc deficiency in man is occurring in the United States from just such a cause. He has noted that throughout the States of North America zinc deficiency is becoming common. High levels of crop production, leaching in acidic soils, superphosphate fertilisation (without the impurities of rock phosphate) and lack of organic manuring are claimed as factors contributing to this. Zinc taken out of the soil is not replaced. Frank zinc deficiency in the human is uncommon and has been diagnosed in Egypt in the malnourished,[18] but low levels of trace element nutrition could contribute to morbidity. Schroeder[22] claims that North Americans have deficient intakes of chromium, manganese and zinc though these deficiencies derive as much from the refining and processing of food as from imbalanced fertilisation of the soil. Zinc forms one of the largest trace metal components of the intracellular compartment and is vital for spermatogenesis, skeletal growth, hair growth and many enzymatic functions within the human body.

Stocks[29] showed that copper deficiency in the soils of North Wales was associated with high incidence of gastric cancer, and patients in this area who died from stomach cancer were eating their own garden vegetables. Voisin[30] also postulated a link between copper deficiency and cancer. These relationships have not been shown to be causal as yet, the evidence is not strong enough. All one can ask is that these factors should be considered. The research world of trace element physiology is a new and expanding one and much is to be expected from it. Only recently Dr. Hurley reported from the University of California, Davis, that transitory deficiency of zinc and magnesium during the pregnancy of rats produced stunted growth and malformations in 90% of the foetuses. Lack of organic fertilisation of contemporary soils could contribute to trace element deficiencies.

Rasmussen[11] reports from America how a survey of 4000 grain samples taken over four years shows a trace element decline. Copper dropped from 2.56 p.p.m. to 0.82 p.p.m. (a 70% decline) and iron dropped from 21 p.p.m. to 15 p.p.m. (a 28.5% decline). In animals, deficiency of copper and iron causes a stress syndrome manifesting in trembling, haemorrhaging and convulsions. Strontium and chromium also showed a decline.

Manurial treatment and plant health
(2) Other nutrients
Schuphan in his *Nutritional Values in Crops and Plants*[23] outlines in detail the many factors that contribute to nutritional quality in crops. They include warmth, light, rainfall, manurial treatments, genetics, harvesting conditions, storage conditions and many other factors. Concentrating on the section of the book which deals with manurial treatments, the following can be noted. Nitrate fertilisation increases total yield of a crop, and crude protein but depresses quality of protein. The Essential Amino Acid index drops for spinach (see Figs. 7.1 and 7.2) for potato (after a sharp initial rise) (Fig. 7.3) and apparently for barley, on adding nitrate. Excess nitrogen fertilisation in celeriac leads to overlargeness and hollow tubers, which show poor keeping properties. Potatoes, cabbage, radish, apples and strawberries react likewise. Benda et al.[3] show too the effects that different nitrogen fertilisers have upon protein quality. (Table 7.1). Comparing urea manuring to liquid ammonia manuring on sugar beet they found the urea gave greater per cent dry matter and a better balance of amino acids in the final product.

Schuphan goes on to show how phosphate fertilisation increases ascorbic acid content but depresses carotene content in lettuce and depresses both vitamins in spinach. Application of potash after a certain point depresses ascorbic acid, carotene, chlorophyll and total acids in spinach. (Fig. 7.4).

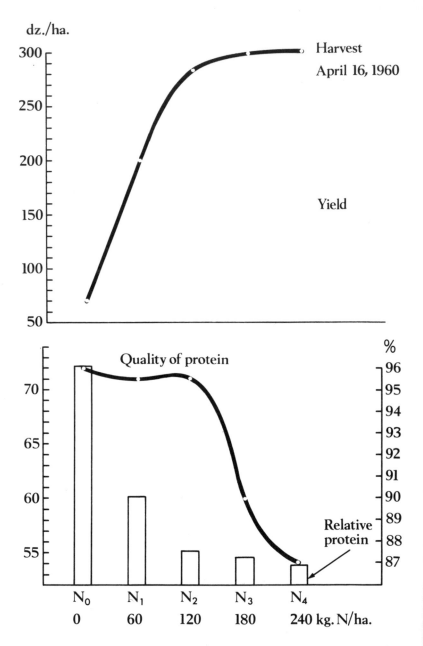

7.1 Effect of nitrogen application on quality of protein in spinach (from Schupan W., *Nutritional Values in Crops and Plants*, Faber, London 1965)

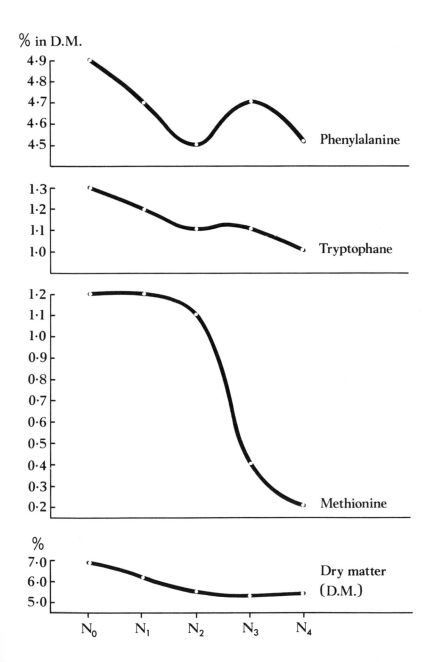

% in D.M.

Phenylalanine

Tryptophane

Methionine

%

Dry matter
(D.M.)

N_0 N_1 N_2 N_3 N_4

7.2 Effect of nitrogen application on certain amino-acids in spinach (from Schupan W., *Nutritional Values in Crops and Plants*, Faber, London 1965)

129

EAA-index for 8 EAA

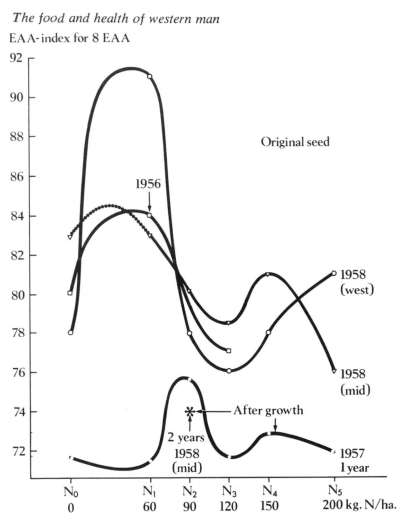

7.3 Effect of nitrogen application on protein quality in the potato (from Schupan, W., *Nutritional Values in Crops and Plants*, Faber, London 1965)

Doring[8] has shown that nitrogen application beyond a certain point depresses vitamin stores in lettuce, spinach, tomato and rye grass. Excessive use of nitrogen can also affect taste qualities and has been shown to produce a metallic taste in tomatoes,[20] and a watery flavoured potato.[2] Excess nitrate fertilisation in spinach can lead to high quantities of nitrate in the vegetable which on storage can reduce to nitrite and poison infants. In Germany 15 infants died over 7 years from high nitrite levels in spinach.[24, 27] Babies carry a foetal haemoglobin and are more susceptible to this form of poisoning than adults, but the spinach has to be heavily fertilised and allowed to stale before being fed to produce this effect.

The effect of organic manures upon nutritional quality has not been studied in such depth and data is hard to find. Scheffer et al.[21] have shown in the case of oats that application of organic

TABLE 7.1
Amino acid content (mg/g of dry matter)
of sugar beet pulp after nitrogen fertilisation

Amino Acid	Treatment with	
	Liquid Ammonia = 2kg Nitrogen	Urea = 2kg Nitrogen
Nitrogen	5.2	10.6
Threonine	0.8	1.10
Glutamic Acid	3.45	6.13
Glycine	1.02	1.18
Cystine	0.45	0.48
Valine	1.34	1.80
Methionine	0.18	0.17
Leucine	1.41	1.69
Lysine	1.35	1.62
Histidine	0.54	0.46

Urea gave greater per cent dry matter
and greater total yield
Source: Benda et al., *J.Sci.Fd.Agric.* 1971. 22:221

manure over and above artificial fertilisation increases the amino-acid content of grain and improves quality. Long-term fertiliser treatments with different kinds of vegetables were carried out in Germany in the years 1936-44.[9, 25] For the most part these experiments showed that combined treatment with farmyard manure + NPK when compared to farmyard manure alone, gave highest yields, best crops, higher protein, carotene, vitamin C and mineral contents, though lower sugars. In dietary studies carried out on these same crops, on adults no differential effect was noted, but on infants a better response was obtained from the combined treatment, farmyard manure + NPK. A better gain in weight was obtained, higher vitamin C and carotene levels in the blood.

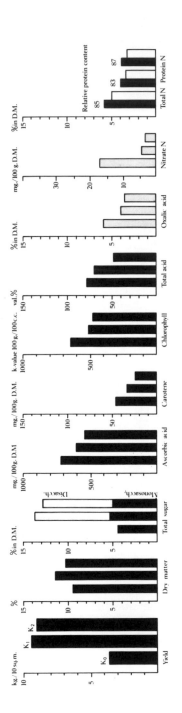

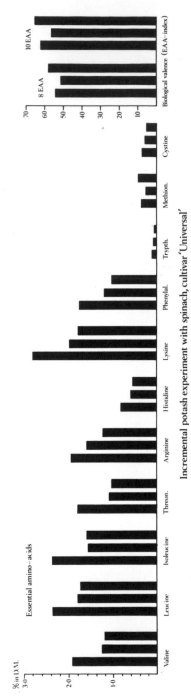

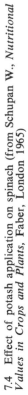

7.4 Effect of potash application on spinach, cultivar 'Universal'
Incremental potash experiment with spinach (from Schupan W., *Nutritional
Values in Crops and Plants*, Faber, London 1965)

Organic manures and animal and human health

Sir Robert McCarrison[14] as far as one is aware is the first and virtually only research worker to have carried out tests on laboratory animals, to define the health difference between compost grown produce and minerally fertilised produce. McCarrison in 1926, analysed growth rates in 54 laboratory rats, divided into

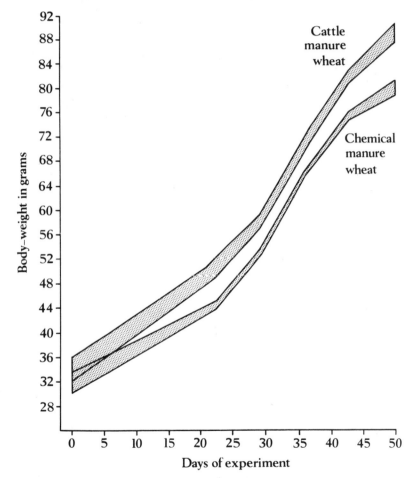

7.5 A comparison of the growth rate of rats fed wheat fertilised differently. Cattle manure wheat came from plots continuously fertilised with farmyard manure at 5 tons/acre. Chemical manure wheat came from plots continuously treated 1 cwt ammonium sulphate/acre, 1 cwt potassium sulphate/acre and 3 cwt superphosphates/ acre.

groups of six. They were fed a basal diet to which was added wheat. The wheat had been taken from plots, some of which had no manure, some had had artificial fertilisers (N. P. and K) and some cattle manure. Figs. 7.5 and 7.6 show the different growth rates of rats on these diets. As will be seen the 'cattle manure' wheat brought about the best performance though the differences are not great. Interestingly, 'no manure' wheat produced perform-

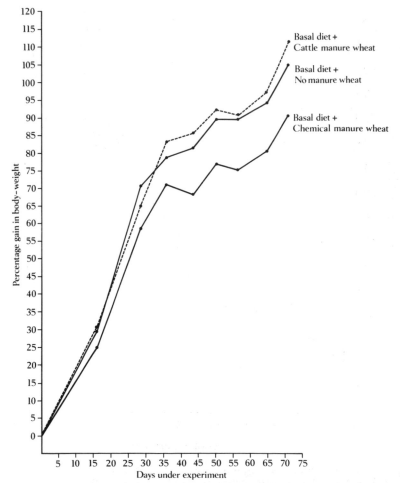

7.6 A comparison of the growth rate of rats fed on wheat fertilised in three different ways (see Fig. 7.5) (from McCarrison R., *Ind. J. Med. Res.*, 1926. 14:351)

ances better than 'chemical manure' which is a little puzzling. McCarrison was only able at that time to carry out certain tests on soil and wheat analysis and one would like to know more concerning the analytical differences between these. In Fig. 7.7 it can be seen that McCarrison put down the nutritional superiority of cattle manure wheat to vitamin A content as he added cod liver oil to chemically manured wheat and growth performance

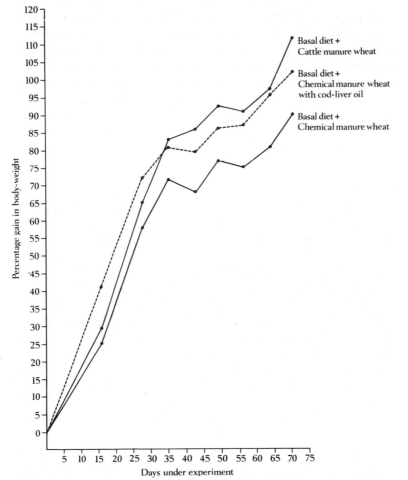

7.7 Growth rate of rats fed on wheat fertilised differently, with cod liver oil added to the diet of one group (see Fig. 7.5) (from McCarrison R., *Ind. J. Med. Res.*, 1926, 14:351).

was almost as good as with the cattle manure rats. Obviously the experiments need repeating under modern conditions and very carefully controlled soil conditions need to confirm these results and analyse the differences.

T. McSheehy of the Pye Research Centre at Haughley is carrying out experiments along similar lines but no results are as yet available.

Scott· Greaves and Scott[25] carried out some breeding tests on mice, using three different wheats taken from the Soil Association farms at Haughley. One wheat sample was from soil artificially fertilised, one sample from soil that had farmyard manure and artificial fertiliser, and a third sample from composted soil. The breeding performance was poor on all three diets compared with a standard diet. Obviously wheat alone is a deficient diet and with such gross deficiency appearing in the mice one could argue that any differences in performance that appeared were meaningless. As the results stand, the mice on the mixed diet fared worst of all.

Protection against cancer

To round up this chapter and the rather scattered data that has been presented, a rather unusual paper that appeared in the *American Journal of Proctology* in February 1961[.6] will be summarised. This paper was written by D. C. Collins, an American surgeon, who was at one time President of the American Society of Proctology. Collins recorded in this paper the spontaneous disappearance of cancer in five patients who had been put on wholefood following the operative removal of the growth. At the operation metastases and spread of the cancer beyond the site of operation had been noted in all five cases. In all patients, when death occurred 21 to 32 years later (from causes other than cancer), post mortem revealed no evidence of cancer whatsoever. Liver metastases had also been present at operation in two of the cases. These had disappeared. The cancers were of colon, caecum and rectum. In each case the patient, post operatively, had eaten consistently of home grown organically raised foods that were not supported by artificial fertiliser or protected by spray. In each case recorded the patient had taken up the practice 'post op.' not practising such gardening before operation. Collins opened his paper thus:

136

This clinical note is written with considerable hesitancy and yet on five different occasions during the past 36 years of practice, I have seen a marvellous phenomenon occur.

He then goes on to detail how biopsies taken at operation

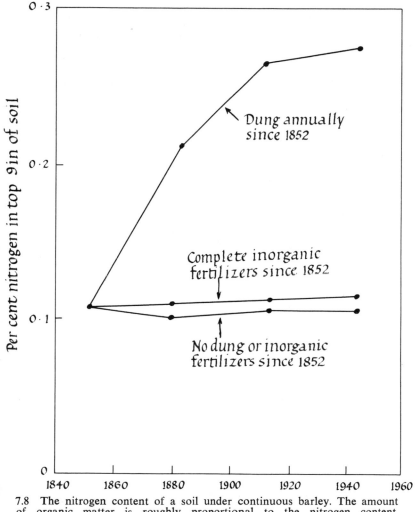

7.8   The nitrogen content of a soil under continuous barley. The amount of organic matter is roughly proportional to the nitrogen content. 0.1% is approximately equivalent to 2% humus (from Jenkinson D., 'Organic Matter in soil', *New Scientist,* Sept. 23, 1965).

revealed carcinoma, how secondaries were carefully noted at the time and how competent pathologists carrying out post mortem examination years later could find no evidence of secondaries (or primary). The results could be explained away by the phenomenon of spontaneous remission. This is known to occur in cancer. The strange point however in these examples is that the disappearance of the cancer was coincident in every case with consumption of organically grown produce. No more dietary details are given other than the fact that the patients raised their vegetable produce in this certain way. Collins queries the possibilities of a plant antibiotic or anticarcinogenic agent in the organically grown vegetables and encourages other surgeons to recommend this 'innocuous' therapy and observe results that might be forthcoming. As far as the author knows no one has taken up this challenge and Dr. Collins has himself now died, but the findings are intriguing.

There is evidence enough that nutritional quality is affected by type of soil fertilisation. What however is needed now is a closer and more scientific appraisal of the differences brought about by chemical and organic manuring and the appropriate laboratory experiments set up to test these differences. It seems clear from the evidence presented in the first part of this chapter that to omit organic manuring is to expose the soil to the possibilities of definite imbalance and deficiency.

This deficiency must affect the health of mankind. The health of the soil as indicated by the level of humus content is dependent on organic manuring. This is shown in Fig. 7.8. It would seem that in the long run the health of the plant grown must also depend upon this humus content, and if this humus content diminishes, as it has been shown to be doing in certain intensively farmed areas, then the health of plant and ultimately man must suffer.

REFERENCES TO CHAPTER 7

1 Ahmed M. K., Jones P.. *Plant Physiol.* 1960, 35: supp. xxix.
2 Bancroft-Wilson J. A., *J. Inst. Corn Agric.,* March 1963, 11:24.
3 Benda P., Dvorak M., Tusl J., *J. Sci. Fd. Agric.* 1971, 22:221.
4 Booth E., *The Grower* 1960. 53:1057.
5 Brown D. A., Albrecht W. A., *Proc. Soil Sci. Soc. Amer.* 1947, 12:342, 1958, 22:303.
6 Collins D. C., *Amer. J. Proctology* 1961, 12:36.

7 Commonwealth Bureau of Soils, *Effects of Fertilisers on Food Crop Quality* 1956-1965, *I General* 819:22, Rothamsted, Harpenden, England, *II Cereals* 819:22:31, *VI Vegetables* 819:22:5.
8 Doring H., *Dtsch. Landwirt* 1961, 12:69 (quoted in 7).
9 Dost F. H., Schuphan W., *Die Ernahrung* 1944, 9:1.
10 Duff R. B., Webley D. M., Scott R. O., *Soil Sci.* 1963, 95:105.
11 *Feedstuffs*, Aug. 9, 1969, p.7.
12 Florescu M., Cernea S., *Inst. Agron 'Dr. Petru. Groza' Cluj.* Lue Stiint. 1961, 17:75 (quoted in 7, VI).
13 Koehler F. E., Albrecht W. A., *Plant and Soil* 1953, 4:336.
14 McCarrison R. 'The effect of manurial conditions on nutritional value of millet and wheat' *Ind. J. Med. Res.* 1926, 14:351.
15 Meschenko V. M., Aleksik V. I., Sabo V. A. *Material y. go mezluiz Sovasch.* 1961, 199 (quoted in 7, I).
16 Novoderzhkina Y. G., *Fiziol. Rast.* 1960, 7:121 (quoted in 7, VI).
17 Parkash V., Bhardwej S. N., *Curr. Sci.* 1964, 33:690.
18 Prasad A. S., Miale A., Favid Z., *J. Lab. Clin. Med.* 1963, 61:537.
19 ——*Zinc Metabolism* Charles C. Thomas, Springfield, Ill. 1965.
20 Saravacos G., Luh B. S., Leonard S. J., *Food Res.* 1958, 23:648.
21 Scheffer E., Kloke A., Alpers H. J., *Z. Pfl Ernahr. Dung* 1957, 78:135. (quoted in 7, II).
22 Schroeder H. A., *Amer. J. Clin. Nut.* 1971, 24:562.
23 Schuphan W., *Qual. Plant Mater. Veg.* 1961, 8:261.
24 ——Dost F. H., Schotola H., *Die Ernahrung* 1940, 5:29, 37.
25 Scott P. P., Greaves J. P., Scott M. G., *Jour. Repro. Fertility* 1960, 1:132.
26 Simon C., *The Lancet* 1966, 1:872.
27 Stancu E., *Inst. Agron 'N. Balescue'* Lue. Stiint 1964, 713:119 (quoted in 7, VI).
28 Stocks P., Davies R. E., *Brit. J. Cancer* 1964, 18:14.
29 Voisin A., *Soil Grass and Cancer*, Crosby & Lockwood, London 1959.
30 ——*Fertiliser Application*, Crosby & Lockwood, London 1965.
31 Wendt H., *Die Ernahrung* 1938, 3:53.

Eight

Health statistics:
America and the U.K.

The health of the British nation from an overall standpoint is poor. Infant mortality has been greatly reduced and infectious diseases curbed but incidence of chronic disease has increased in every age group over 25. The major chronic diseases; cancer, heart disease, bronchitis, rheumatism and arthritis have all increased in prevalence within the population, and this after excluding the factors of population ageing and population increase. Minor chronic disease; obesity, dental caries, mental illness, diabetes, intestinal diseases etc. have also shown a rise in incidence. It is well known that more people are surviving into middle age, the population is ageing as infection in infancy and youth is curbed, but amongst those that survive a higher incidence than ever of chronic ill-health is being recorded.

It is with this fact in mind that one cannot in any way agree with the Minister of Health when in a report on the nation's health, he states that the health record of the country continues to improve in many ways! On the contrary the health of the country continues to deteriorate in many ways. Expectation of life for the middle-aged English male is virtually the same in 1968 as in 1950. It actually fell two points in 1963 (Table 8.1). This despite the huge increase in anti-infective agents such as antibiotics to curb our pneumonias etc. The middle-aged American male has actually dropped his life expectancy from 27.5 years at the age of 45 to 25.8 years. He is now expected to die earlier! This cannot be said to be the golden age of medicine. These figures also do not reveal the vast area of morbidity which modern drugs support and palliate as we move into old age. Is this really the best we can do?

140

Mortality

Heart and circulatory disease is our number one killer accounting for 37% of deaths. Add to this the 14% of deaths due to cerebro-vascular accident and about 50% of deaths can be said to be due to 'blood vessel disease'. Cancer of all types accounts for 20% of deaths.

It is revealing also to look at death in the productive years of life, 15 to 64. In this age group:

Cancer accounts for	...	29%	of deaths
Circulatory disease	...	27%	of deaths
Accident and violence	...	17%	of deaths
Cerebrovascular disease	...	6%	of deaths

Figs. 8.1 and 8.2 show how patterns of mortality have changed over the past 50 years. Figs. 8.3 and 8.4 show how heart disease

8.1 Leading causes of death 1970 (from *Annual Report of Chief Medical Officer of Ministry of Health,* 1971)

has increased in incidence within the population. In 1970, 80,844 men died from ischemic heart disease and 28,700 of these men were between the ages of 40 and 64, if not in their prime of life at least their most productive years. From 1930, heart disease has almost doubled its death toll each decade and has now reached a point where 20% of all middle aged men can expect to develop clinical symptoms of heart disease during their middle years of life! Obesity, hypertension, smoking and high blood cholesterol

y
The food and health of western man

levels are factors which increase the risk of a man developing heart disease.

Cancer of the lung has risen at a rate of increase not far behind heart disease (see Fig. 8.3) and the increase has been fast over the past ten years. Women too are now smoking far more than was customary. This disease also strikes middle-age. In 1970, 25,840

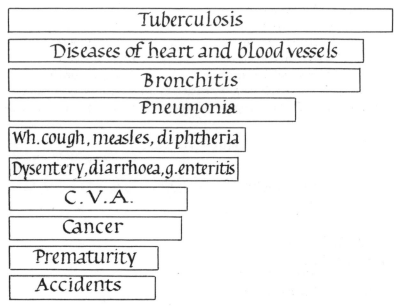

8.2   The commonest causes of death in 1900

men died from cancer of the lung, 50% of these were between the ages of 40 and 64. The peak of mortality reached for this disease in Great Britain amongst middle aged men is almost three times higher than in Canada and twice as high as in Scandinavia. Expectation of life is worse in fact for the middle aged man in Britain than most other European countries.[14]

Fig. 8.3 shows changing trends in mortality for other diseases over the past ten years. Bronchopneumonia is increasing its rate but as it is often the cause of death in the very old, whose total numbers are increasing also, too much attention should not be paid to the rise. Cancers other than cancer of the lung are only very slowly rising, a fact that tends to disprove the theory that our

142

total carcinogenic (cancer causing) environment is becoming more potent. Some cancers are decreasing in importance as cause of death (stomach, intestine, rectum) others are increasing, though slowly (breast, ovary, pancreas). Their increase is possible to

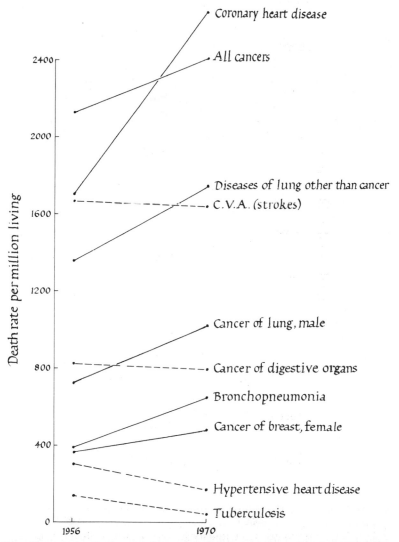

8.3   Changes in death rates for some of the commoner diseases 1956-1970 (from Registrar General's *Statistical Review,* 1970)

143

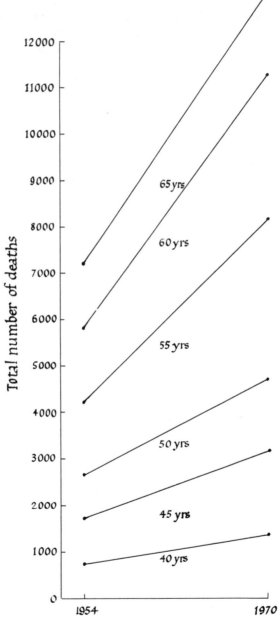

8.4 Rise in death rates for coronary heart disease at different age levels amongst U.K. population, male (from Registrar General's *Statistical Review,* 1970)

explain again on the basis of an aging population. Against this apparent plateau reached in total cancer, must be put the fact that successful surgery and radiotherapy have forestalled death for many. These therapies are increasing in their efficiency and *may therefore hide a real increase in incidence* of total cancers at the present time.

Expectation of life
For the infant, life holds out much better prospects now than was the case in 1900. For the middle aged man this is not so. Tables 8.1 and 8.2 compare life expectancy in England and Wales and in America. In America, life expectancy for the infant has increased

TABLE 8.1
Expectation of Life in England and Wales 1930-1968[14]

Age	Males				Females			
	1930-2	1948-50	1963	1968	1930-2	1948-50	1963	1968
35	33.9	36.0	36.1	36.5	36.9	40.1	41.3	42.0
45	25.5	27.0	26.8	27.2	28.3	30.9	31.9	32.7
55	17.9	18.8	18.5	18.8	20.2	22.4	23.1	23.9
65	11.3	12.3	11.8	12.0	13.1	14.6	15.1	15.9

TABLE 8.2
Expectation of Life in America 1900-1968

Age	Males				Females			
	1900	1930	1957	1968	1900	1930	1957	1968
0	46.3	58	66.3	66.6	48.3	61.6	72.5	74.0
45	25.6		27.5	25.8	31.7		36.8	32.5
65	11.5	11.7	12.6	12.8	12.2	12.8	15.3	16.3

an average of 20 years if he is a boy, 24 if a girl, but on the other hand for the middle-aged hardly at all if he is a man and one year if a woman! In England and Wales, since 1930 life expectancy has increased two years for males of 45 and one year for males of 55 hardly an impressive increase in health prospects. Between the years of 1950 and 1963 there was actually a *decrease* in life expectancy for the middle-aged English male![6, 10] As regards men the civil service estimate the health of their male members by stating that a man of 25 has just over a one in three chance of death

The food and health of western man

or premature retirement before achieving his pension at 60![10]

Britain's health is less than other European countries and Table 8.3 shows comparisons between countries. Death rates for the middle aged man are compared between European nations. Rates are almost twice as high in Scotland as in Sweden and in fact Britain comes near the bottom of the 'European tables'. A man in Norway has a twice better chance of surviving from 65 to 85 as a man in England.[14] The woman again fares better. France

TABLE 8.3
Death Rates per 1000 in the years of age
45-64 for some developed countries 1963[14]

Ages	45-49	50-54	55-59	60-64
Sweden	4.0	6.2	10.9	18.8
Holland	4.4	7.5	12.8	20.6
Canada	5.7	9.4	15.4	24.1
Italy	5.8	9.3	15.5	25.0
England, Wales	5.4	9.5	17.1	28.8
Scotland	7.2	11.9	21.0	34.0

only marginally better than Britain in 1950, is now quite a lot healthier as regards her prospects. Why this difference? Cancer of the lung and bronchitis have a higher incidence in this country than other European countries and we also seem to be suffering more middle-aged heart disease than foreign countries apart from America. These are the main reasons.

Morbidity
To an extent true health is not measured by what we die from but what we suffer from when we live. Morbidity, the state of disease of the living, is dependent for its findings upon the accurate measurement of disease and health. Unless one can quantitate some factor, and this factor represents disease or health in some respect, little can be achieved. Disagreements often exist in medicine as to which factor should be measured and what the measurement means. An example is the haemoglobin level that defines iron deficiency anaemia. Controversy exists as to which level of haemoglobin should be chosen in surveys to represent anaemia

146

and further to this some commentators consider the haemoglobin level now irrelevant and would prefer to rely upon the more inaccessible measurements of serum iron or stainable marrow stores. What at first appears as a simply defined problem often proves more complicated.

Diabetes is another frequently assessed abnormality and here the problem is more complex. Diabetes is, in middle age, a disease of gradual onset characterised by rising blood sugar and the appearance of sugar in the urine. But urine sugar is an inexact method of screening for diabetes which method has now been proved to miss the detection of a large number of cases.[7] Blood sugar is a more exact means of identification but the problem exists as to which level should be taken as diagnostic. In any survey a broad spectrum of resultant levels presents itself from the lowest blood sugar to the highest. An arbitrary point is taken as the 'cut-off' level above which diabetes is diagnosed, below which it is not. Variation unfortunately exists between scientists as to 'cut-off' levels chosen and different surveys lack standardisation. Rheumatism and arthritis are examples of conditions where no 'blood sugar level' exists and diagnosis depends on the patient's description of his symptoms as much as any measurable sign. Such conditions become difficult to assess and in this case estimates either rely upon X-ray changes, again difficult to standardise, or fall back upon subjective reports of pain, stiffness or swelling. Errors in measurement must therefore abound regarding such conditions and have to be borne in mind when statistics are used.

Few accurate population surveys of morbidity have been carried out where good data are available. Such surveys of total disease are expensive, time consuming and need many staff to organise them. The National Centre for Health Statistics[15] in America have established assessments of chronic illness from interview surveys and a commission on Chronic Illness was set up by the American Medical Association and other bodies in the United States to assess chronic illness between 1949 and 1956 in a large city, Baltimore[3] and a rural area, Hunterdon County, New Jersey, U.S.A.[4] As this was a very full and carefully worked study much information is used from it in the following pages. On comparison of the findings with English statistics, quite close correlation is noted, suggesting that chronic illness in the two countries may be of similar magnitude.

147

Prevalence of chronic illness

Table 8.4 compares the prevalence of disease found in the American surveys at Baltimore[3] and Hunterdon County[4] with various surveys on individual disease carried out in this country.

TABLE 8.4
Incidence of chronic disease in the total population, in America and in United Kingdom

Disease	Separate studies carried out on individual diseases in United Kingdom. Percentage incidence in adult population.		Baltimore City U.S.A.[3] 1950-56 Percentage incidence	Hunterdon County[4] U.S.A. 1950-56 Percentage incidence
Obesity			12.8	15.5
Diseases of female genital tract			13.3	*28
Heart disease			9.6	11.8
Hypertension	7[11]		6.6	11.8
Psychiatric illness	6.2[11]		6.6	13
Osteoarthritis	6[8]	12[9]	7.5	8.3
Rheumatoid arthritis	2[12]		1.7	
General aches, pains	33[8]			••33
Peptic ulcer	5.9[5]	10.2[21]	3.6	3.4
Dyspepsia	31[5]	35[21]		
Diabetes	•••12[2]	4[7]	2.7	1.0
Anaemia	10[11]		2.6	
Hernia			3.6	3.0
Tumours (benign and malignant)			5.4	6.1
Varicose veins			4.3	4.7
Skin				8.7
Thyroid disease			2.4	4.0
Deafness			2.0	2.8
Bronchitis	3[11]			0.8
Urine infections	1.4[11]		1.8	2.8
Prostate disease			4.4	10

* This figure includes disorders of menstruation, menopause and the female genital tract.
** This survey was carried out in Tecumseh, Michigan.
*** This survey in Bedford included testing blood glucose tolerance curves as well as screening for urine sugar.

Quite close correlation is noted. Where there is discrepancy it is generally due to the contrast between a more thorough survey (e.g. the Bedford diabetes survey) and one less thorough. In Baltimore and Hunterdon County tests were made for sugar in the urine only. This would seem to indicate that the findings for diabetes are on the whole an underestimate rather than an overestimate.

The most significant finding in Hunterdon County was that 86% of the population were suffering from one or more chronic illnesses, 65% in Baltimore. Table 8.5 shows how this varied according to age. In the 15-34 age group only 31% suffered one or more substantial chronic conditions. In the over 65 age group

TABLE 8.5
Percentage of persons with chronic substantial
disease by age[3]

Age	Percentage of persons with one or more :	
	Chronic conditions	Substantial chronic conditions
-15	29.2	17.4
15-34	63.5	31.0
35-64	85.8	65.9
65+	95.4	85.2
TOTAL %	64.9	44.4

85% suffered a substantial chronic condition. The surprising frequency of chronic illness in the young and indeed the old is explained perhaps by the completeness of the survey. Many disease categories were included from dental disease and obesity to psychoneurosis, kidney disease and skin disease. Tables 8.6, 8.7, 8.8, 8.9 show which diseases were common at which age group.

TABLE 8.6
Diseases common in the 15-24 age group, and of
less serious prognosis. Hunterdon County[4]

Disease	*% Incidence*
Mental, psychoneurotic, personality disorders	17.8
Dental disease	15.1
Menstrual disorders	9.4
Skin diseases	6.1
Refractive errors, eye	5.8
Hay fever	5.1
Abdominal hernia	4.3

For instance amongst the young commonest chronic conditions were psychoneurotic disorders (17%), dental disease (15%), menstrual disorders (9%), skin disease (6%) and hay fever (5%). Amongst

149

the over 65s, the conditions are more serious and include heart disease, arthritis and cancer. Substantial conditions (as estimated in Table 8.5) include any disease which interfered with or limited the patient's activities. Such conditions therefore included, heart

TABLE 8.7
Diseases common in the 25-44 age group. Percentage incidence in age group concerned.
Hunterdon County[4]

Disease	% Incidence
Female genital diseases	36.4
Refractive errors, eye	34.6
Obesity	24.3
Hypertension	16.1
Dental disease	15.9
Mental, psychoneurotic and personality disorders	13.6
Skin disease	11.1
Thyroid disease	8.3

*Categorised as a disease of serious prognosis.

TABLE 8.8
Diseases common in the 45-64 age group. Percentage incidence in age group concerned.
Hunterdon County[4]

Disease	% Incidence
Refractive errors, eye	51.7
Female genital disease	42.0
*Hypertension	27.0
*Arthritis	23.8
Dental disease	23.6
Obesity	20.9
*Prostate disease	18.2
*Heart disease	18.1
Varicose veins	13.7

*Categorised as a disease of serious prognosis

diseases, cancer, kidney disease, arthritis, psychosis, psychoneurosis, sinusitis, gall bladder disease but not deafness, varicose veins, hay fever, skin disease etc.

Out of this large mass of chronic illness, disablement was small. Only 4% of all subjects were limited in performance of daily duties, and they were mostly the older patients. 5-8% had slight limitations and 90% of conditions imposed no limitations. Females

150

on the whole were more susceptible to chronic illness than the males and there were no females over 65 who were free of disease. 86% of all conditions found were considered continuous with no remissions from the disease expected.

Perhaps the most disheartening of all news concerns the

TABLE 8.9
Diseases common in 65+ age group. Percentage
incidence in age group concerned.
Hunterdon County[4]

Disease	% Incidence
*Heart disease	64.6
*Prostate disease	50.5
Refractive errors, eye	39.7
*Arthritis	36
*General arteriosclerosis	29.1
*Eye disease	14.3
Dental disease	14.0
Respiratory disease (bronchitis)	14.0
*Malignant neoplasms	12.0

*Categorised as a disease
of serious prognosis

TABLE 8.10
Degree of preventability at time of interview of diseases
found in population of Hunterdon County[4]

Unpreventable at our present state of knowledge	Partially preventable; possible to prevent disease reaching an advanced stage	Totally preventable
Most:	A lot of:	Some:
Neoplasms (cancer)	Digestive disease	Obesity
Eye disease	Dental disease	Dental disease
	Mental disorders	
A lot of:	Obesity	A fraction of:
Heart disease	Infective disease	Mental disorder
Circulatory disease		Skin disease
Arthritis	Some:	
Ear disease	Skin diseases	
	Allergies	
Some:		
Allergic conditions		
Respiratory disease		
TOTAL		
*PERCENTAGE 40	33	6

* 21% of diseases could not definitely be allotted to any category.

151

preventability of diseases found. Despite the good health education and available medical services few of the chronic illnesses were truly preventable. The authors, as is shown in Table 8.10, classify only 6% of conditions as truly so. The 6% includes some obesity and dental disease and a small fraction of the mental and skin disease. This is perhaps a pessimistic impression and the authors categorise 21% of disease into a category of undecided preventability. About these diseases the authors prefer not to commit themselves, but it speaks of a certain helplessness in medicine today concerning many chronic illnesses which seem to defeat modern therapy. True preventive medicine is in fact yet a long way from realisation.

No such surveys as these exist in Britain at the present moment though certain attempts have been made on a small scale to detect undiscovered disease. J. M. Last[11] in a survey within a general practice in East London estimated the frequency of certain nine diseases and found a fair quantity of disease below the tip of the clinical iceberg. These findings have been tentatively used for the purpose of assessing morbidity in the general population. Last's figures have been extrapolated.[16]

As a result it is said there are unrecognised 2-3 million hypertensives, 300,000 women with untreated urinary infection, the same number with untreated rheumatoid arthritis, 1.3 million in need of psychiatric care, 400,000 with undiscovered diabetes and 700,000 undiscovered bronchitics in need of treatment. The number of people with these seven diseases only, tolerating ill-health totals five million or one in 10 of the population.

Dr. Innes Pearse and I. H. Crocker in the Peckham Experiment[19] recount how in Peckham before the war in the first truly family Health Centre to be founded in this country, 3066 individuals were medically examined between 1935 and 1939. 90% of individuals as a result were classified as suffering from some identifiable disorder or disease. In Hunterdon County the figure was 86%. In Peckham only 26% of the population were actually suffering from their disease, another 8% were under treatment and 64% were unaffected by their disease. Again conditions diagnosed ranged over such disorders as dental disease, digestive disorders, iron and vitamin deficiency, to such serious diseases as nephritis, haematuria and cancer.

General practitioner surveys[13] show which diseases bring the patient most often to the doctor. Table 8.11 shows the most frequent of these, the common cold heading the list. Diseases which account for most of chronic illness seen by general practitioners are in order: bronchitis, arthritis and rheumatism and psychoneurotic disorders. Muscular rheumatism, fibrositis and sciatica account for the body of rheumatic complaints, the rest being due to osteo-arthritis and back pain.

TABLE 8.11
Diseases with the highest consulting rates[13]

Disease	Number of patients consulting per 1000
Common cold	81.1
Arthritis, rheumatism	64.9
Bronchitis	62.3
Psychoneurotic disorders	45.7
Influenza	38.2
Tonsillitis	35.2
Pharyngitis	28.3
Disorders of menstruation	24.1
Gastroenteritis, colitis	22.2
Disorders of stomach, other.	21.5

TABLE 8.12
Causes for admission to hospital for those between years 45-64.
Spells per 10,000 population in England and Wales 1962[14]

Medical

Male		Female	
Heart (coronary)	49	Stroke	15
Bronchitis	34	Heart (coronary)	14
Pneumonia	19	Skin	13
T.B.	17	Bronchitis	11
Hypertension	13	Psychoneurosis	11

Surgical

Male		Female	
Hernia	59	Prolapse uterus	38
Peptic ulcer	39	Cancer breast	22
Cancer, lung	33	Gall bladder	22
Eye disease	18	Varicose veins	23
Head injury	18	Fibroid of uterus	19
Urinary disease	17	Eye disease	17
Prostate	13	Urinary disease	15

Disease and middle age

Most serious chronic health starts in middle age and therefore it is instructive to examine trends of illness in this age group. Table 8.12 shows what diseases take the patients, in the middle age group of 45-64, most frequently to hospital in the U.K. More men are admitted to the medical wards at this age than women. The women make up for it later. Heart disease and bronchitis are the main causes for men. Surgically, hernia, peptic ulcer and cancer of the lung predominate for the men and prolapsed uterus, cancer of the breast, gall bladder disease and varicose veins for the women. Peptic ulcer is seen still to figure largely in male surgical diseases even though admissions are on the decrease.

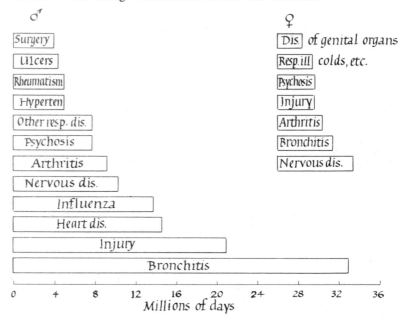

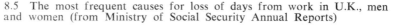

8.5 The most frequent causes for loss of days from work in U.K., men and women (from Ministry of Social Security Annual Reports)

Hospital admissions can only be accepted as rough guides to actual incidence of disease as so many factors operate to influence them. However, increases in admission rates over the past ten years are as follows:

		approximately
Heart disease	... ...	150%
Bronchitis, Cancer of lung	...	100%
Stroke, Cervicitis	... ...	100%
Asthma, Leukemia	... ...	100%
Osteoarthritis	... ...	70%
Urinary disease	... ...	50%

Main causes for ill-health in this age group are shown by Figure 8.5 where bronchitis, injury, heart disease, influenza, psychoneurotic disease and arthritis head the list of conditions that take a man off work. For women psychoneurotic disease, bronchitis, arthritis and injury are in the lead. The number of consultations a man in middle age makes to his doctor (Table 8.13) increases in frequency

TABLE 8.13
Annual General Practitioner consulting rates
in Barrow 1960-61[14]

Age	Male		Female	
	Consultations per year	Drug cost s. d.	Consultations per year	Drug cost s. d.
-15	5.0	16 3	5.5	19 4
16-45	3.8	16 3	5.7	29 4
46-65	5.8	36 7	5.7	39 7
66+	5.0	32 8	8.7	50 9

and expense compared to youth, indicating longer or more expensive treatment. The expense is in fact double what it averages in the 15-45 age group. Interestingly it falls off in old age amongst the men, the women taking over and taking most time with the doctor.

In his forties the average man is off work for two weeks, but in his mid-fifties this doubles to four weeks, rising at 60 to seven weeks. Men incapacitated from work for over three months make up 7% of the labour force by age of 55 but 10% at 60 years of age.[14]

In Fig. 8.6 an attempt has been made to illustrate the frequency of substantial disease in the middle-aged population. For the sake of clarity it has been impossible to show diseases overlapping which they will do obviously in real life, and certain diseases are therefore omitted, such as haemorrhoids and hernia in men, and rheumatic disease in women. Nevertheless it has been assessed[14] that in middle age:

1 in 4 men will suffer chronic bronchitis
1 in 5 men will develop heart disease
1 in 12 men will have a peptic ulcer
1 in 4 men will develop cancer, of whom
1 in 30 will die from cancer of the lung
1 in 35 will die from cancer of the stomach

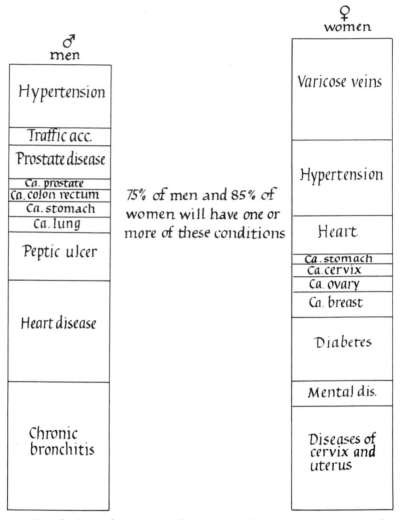

8.6 Distribution of some of the more serious diseases amongst the elderly and middle ages (from Logan R. F., *Roy. Soc. Health Jour.*, 1967, 87:298)

For women:

    1 in 4 will be regularly attending the G.P. with a chronic disorder

    1 in 8 will be liable to diabetes

    1 in 5 will develop cancer, of which

    1 in 20 will die from cancer of the breast

    1 in 35 will develop cancer of the ovaries

What the future holds

The future is not altogether promising as regards chronic illness in this country for several reasons. These are as follows:

(1) Total population is rising.
(2) The population is ageing.
(3) No real breakthrough has occurred in the treatment of these chronic diseases in the last 15 years, and certainly not in prevention of them.
(4) Actual increase in incidence of these diseases seems to be occurring independent of population changes. Certainly this is so for heart disease and cancer of the lung.

Fig. 8.7 shows how the population has changed in Britain since 1851. The number of people over 65 has risen fast and risen

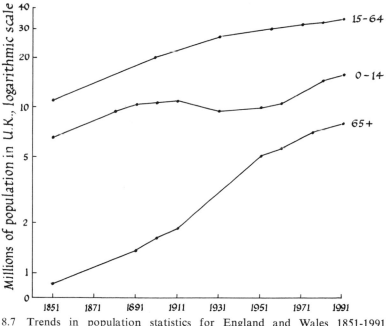

8.7 Trends in population statistics for England and Wales 1851-1991 (from *Old Age*, Office of Health Economics, 1968 and Registrar General's *Statistical Review*)

as a proportion of the whole. Population increases are difficult to forecast with accuracy. Certain economic restrictions of late in this country may have an effect in reducing birth rate and so reducing total population. The rise therefore shown in Fig. 8.7 for those between 0 and 14 may not take place to the extent shown. However with improved maternity care, obstetrics and paediatrics more people are surviving into middle age. Women are improving their expectancy of life into very old age (though only slightly) and the total number of people living over 65 years of age is expected to rise according to statisticians from a present 5.9 million to between seven and eight million in 1991.[18] This alone will increase chronic disease in the community. *The position is worse in America*[20] where faster population increases and greater drift of population into old age are expected to raise chronic illness very considerably (see Table 8.14). The increase in number of people over 45 with major limitation of activity is expected to increase by 50%. The increase

TABLE 8.14
Increases expected in chronic illness in America between
1961 and 1981 in older age group[20]

	Percentage increase	
	45 yrs +	65 yrs +
Those with one or more chronic illnesses	31.7	50.8
Those with major limitations of activity	47.4	55.1
Increase in heart disease	37.5	50.5
Increase in Diabetes	37.2	49.0
Increase in Arthritis and Rheumatism	35.7	50.8
Increase in Deafness	42.5	54.5

in numbers of those over 65 with a chronic illness is expected to increase also by 50%. These figures in absolute numbers mean *an increase of 10 million persons over 45 and 6.5 million over 65, with chronic illness.* These increases are merely from population increases and population ageing. No account has been taken of 'real' increase in incidence in any one disease. They are therefore underestimates.

Heart disease and lung disease definitely show real increase. It is more difficult with other conditions to be accurately sure. *The American National Health Survey*[15] *however in examining incidence of chronic disease in America have found real increases taking place in every age group* (Table 8.15). These figures are recorded by National Health Surveys. There is no real reason to expect the situation to be different in the U.K. In this country the only
158

comparable survey of health that exists for comparison is the return from the Ministry of Social Security showing days lost from work via claims for sickness benefit. Fig. 8.8 shows the trend. 330 million days of certified sickness absence are recorded for the

TABLE 8.15

Increase in frequency of chronic illness in the population over 4 years from National Health Surveys of America[15, 20]

Age	Year 1962-63	1963-64	1964-65	1965-66
Under 17	20.1	20.6	21.4	22.4
17-24	37.7	38.8	39.5	43.2
25-44	52.4	53.1	55.2	59.2
45-64	64.3	65.4	66.2	70.6
65+	81.2	82.3	83.4	85.2

year. This is an understatement for reasons that short spells are not recorded (under 3 days). 75% of married women opt out of national insurance and professional staff and, most importantly of all, housewives are not recorded in this assessment.

The Office of Health Economics analyses these trends in two publications[17] and assesses how much real ill-health this represents.

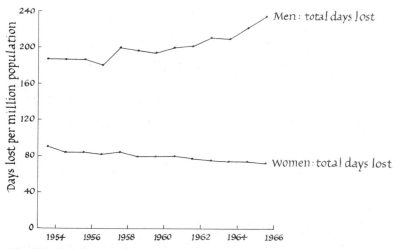

8.8 Working days lost amongst insured population, England and Wales, 1954-1966 (from Ministry of Social Security Annual Reports)

The food and health of western man

It would seem that alongside other data presented in this chapter we have here substantial confirmation of the fact that chronic illness is increasing in the community in a serious manner.

Summary

Mortality and morbidity have been analysed and contrasted with regard to the health of this country. Mortality is rising from heart disease and cancer of the lung. These two diseases account for the poor life expectancy of the middle aged man in America and Britain today. But more importantly a huge area of morbidity and chronic sickness exists within the community shown by the evidence above. Is this a state of health to be proud over? Do we sit back and pat our Health Service or anyone else on the back in such circumstances? It has been shown in careful studies that 60-80% of the population are suffering from one or more chronic illnesses. The prevalence will rise inevitably as the population ages, but apart from this there is evidence from many quarters of a real increase in frequency of chronic disease distinct from that produced by population changes. This is the alarming fact and particularly so as medicine has no current means of preventing this. Health will decline until these illnesses can be prevented.

REFERENCES TO CHAPTER 8

1 Annual Report of Chief Officer, Ministry of Health *On the State of Public Health* 1970, H.M.S.O. 1971.
2 Butterfield W. J., *Proc. Roy. Soc. Med.* 1964, 57:195.
3 *Chronic Illness in the United States.* Vol. III *Chronic Illness in a Large City* by the Commission on Chronic Illness, Harvard Univ. Press, Cambridge U.S.A. 1957.
4 *Chronic Illness in the United States.* Vol. IV *Chronic Illness in a Rural Area* Tressell R. E., Ellinson J., Harvard Univ. Press, Cambridge U.S.A. 1957.
5 Doll R., Jones F. A., Buckatzsch M. M., *Spec. rep. ser. Med. Res. Coun.* 276, 1951.
6 ——Hill A. B., *Brit. Med. J.* 1964, 1:1460.
7 Keen H., *Proc. Roy. Soc. Med.* 1964, 57:200.
8 Kellgren J. H., Lawrence J. S., Aitken Swan J., *Ann Rheum. Dis.* 1953, 12:5.
9 —,—*Ann. Rheum. Dis.* 1956, 15:1.
10 *The Lancet* 1964, 1:1201.
11 Last J. M., *The Lancet* 1963, 2:28.
12 Lawrence, J. S., *Ann. Rheum. Dis.* 1961, 20:11.
13 Logan W. P. D., Cushion A. A., General Register Office. *Studies on Medical and Population Subjects* No. 14, Vol. 1 (general) H.M.S.O. 1958.

[14] Logan R. F. L., *Roy Soc. Health J.* 1967. 87:298.
[15] National Health Survey U.S. Publ. Health Serv. series 1600:10 Nos. 5, 13, 25, 37.
[16] Office Health Economics publication *New Frontiers of Health*, O.H.E. London 1964.
[17] Office Health Economics publication *Work Lost through Sickness* and *Off Sick*, O.H.E. London 1965 and 1971.
[18] Office Health Economics publication *Old Age*, O.H.E. London 1968.
[19] Pearse I. H., Crocker L. H. *The Peckham Experiment*, Allen & Unwin London 1943.
[20] Twaddle A. C., *J. Chron. Dis.* 1968, 21:417.
[21] Weir R. D., Backett M., *Gut* 1968, 9:75.

Nine

Heart disease

Nutritionally speaking heart disease is caused by eating too rich a diet. The three components of our diet which are at fault are fat, sugar and refined carbohydrate.

In the scientific world it is the nature of the scientific attitude to analyse a problem by a process of fragmentation, to break down a problem to its component parts and carry out research upon these single factors. Complexity is a challenge to the research worker in such a case· and must be reduced to simplicity. Heart disease, as with many chronic degenerative diseases, is caused and influenced by *many factors*. To argue that only one factor is operative, or all-important is short sighted and illogical. It is rather akin to saying only one factor in the temperament goes to make a politician and all other parts of the human character are unimportant. Our hearts and blood vessels, albeit thickened and hardened with atherosclerotic plaques, are integrated components of our human body. They are, therefore, acted upon by physical, dietary, hormonal and psychological factors throughout their lifetime. Each one of these factors must affect the status and health of these structures. Coronary heart disease, as is the case with most chronic degenerative diseases, is aetiologically a multi-factorial disease. Many factors in the western world contribute to this disease. They are as follows:

Obesity and overnutrition[15, 37, 61]
High consumption of animal fats[45, 47, 55]
High consumption of sucrose, and refined carbohydrates[72, 94, 96]
Cigarette smoking[18, 37]
Lack of exercise[68, 69]
Hardness or softness of water[14]

162

Trace element deficiencies, e.g. chromium, vanadium[65]

Psychological stress[22, 27, 84]

Constitutional body type including:

    (a)   body build[37]

    (b)   sex, male or female[40]

    (c)   other genetic factors[40]

Associated diseases such as hypertension, diabetes, gout, hypercholesterolemia.

The first eight factors together with the associated diseases listed are environmentally related to 'western civilisation'. The 'coronary type' who drinks hard, eats hard and works hard is no caricature. He exists, though a simplification. With so many factors affecting a chronic disease and others no doubt as yet undiscovered it becomes difficult and perhaps illogical to isolate merely one factor as causally important. It would be a research worker's dream come true, if such were possible. The position is not made easier by the fact that every research worker in the field believes that this particular dream will come true, that his particular factor will prove to be the causal factor. Hence the position at the present time. One professor champions sugar, another champions fat. A third relates to psychological factors and a fourth is conducting work upon trace elements or hardness of the water. Each in his own turn must prove his hypothesis, for this is the nature of science, at the expense of the other, each forgetting that the human body is more complex than a laboratory bench might suggest and absorbs and reacts to many different environmental influences at one time. Naturally the laboratory bench is contributory to the greater understanding but let us retain the accent on the 'greater understanding'. The eyes of the research worker are often a little short-sighted.

The nutritional factors incriminated so far with regard to coronary heart disease are fats, sugar and refined carbohydrate, and obesity and overnutrition in general. The work upon these at the present time will be summarised.

Fats

Fats are classified as hard or soft, respectively animal or vegetable, saturated and unsaturated. Termed hard and soft according to the temperature at which they melt, animal fats found in meat, milk, eggs and butter are more solid at room temperature than the unsaturated oils found in seeds, nuts and fish. Examples of these unsaturated oils are corn oil, soy bean oil, cotton seed oil, sunflower seed oil, and fats found in walnuts, almonds and fish. Olive oil is intermediate between hard and soft. The hard fats, the animal fats are deemed harmful.

Ingestion of animal fats leads to a rise in blood cholesterol. Cholesterol is one of the constituents, in fact the principal constituent, of the atherosclerotic plaque. This plaque is the name given to the thickening that takes place along the wall of the large arteries which in turn gives rise to occlusion of blood vessels and leads to coronary thrombosis, cerebral vascular disease and peripheral arterial disease. Cholesterol is itself a lipid (or fat) component of the blood which is invariably raised in patients prone to coronary thrombosis.[64, 78]

One might reasonably ask as to why animal fat, a food that has been eaten by men in Britain and America over many centuries, should in this day and age be designated harmful. For the fat off the joint in days gone by was considered tasty and desirable and joints were fattier than those eaten nowadays. Butter and cheese have also long been eaten within these shores.

Two points are immediately important here. Firstly fat consumption has risen over the past 70 years. This was outlined in the first chapter. Particularly has the consumption increased of milk, butter and eggs. Butter itself contains a potent cholesterol raising factor, myristic acid. Secondly the meat of today contains far more saturated fat (and mono-unsaturated short chain fats) than the meat of yesteryear.[44] M. A. Crawford[13] has shown that the modern high fat carcass produced by intensive husbandry may have 25-30% fat and only 50-55% lean. On the other hand a cow free to select its own food and range over the land has been shown to have a carcass fat of 3.9% and a lean tissue mass of 79%. This is a huge difference. Thirdly as will be mentioned later, there is the reality of interaction and potentiation. Sucrose can potentiate fat in the raising of cholesterol within the human blood.

Some of the experimental evidence linking fat consumption to coronary heart disease is as follows. A large number of experiments on different sorts of animals have clearly shown that atheroma can be induced in a relatively short time by artificially raising the blood cholesterol. This can best be done by feeding the animals a diet containing cholesterol and saturated fat.[60] The correlation between blood cholesterol levels and coronary heart disease in such wide ranging studies as that at Framingham, Massachusetts, confirm that this serum factor is a significant one in the production of heart disease.[7, 78]

Many animal experiments now confirm that feeding cholesterol and hard fat causes high blood cholesterol and atherogenesis. The feeding of poly-unsaturated fatty acids counters this rise. This evidence has been summarised by Malmros in his review and elsewhere.[60, 64]

Many foods raise blood fat levels and, since the time when the importance of cholesterol was first outlined in the pathogenesis of heart disease, foods have been variously incriminated in heart disease. For instance a meal of cornflakes, milk and sugar, eggs, bacon and coffee is a meal designed to raise blood fats. Every one of the substances mentioned, excepting cornflakes, has been shown to raise blood cholesterol, even coffee.[33, 54] Katz, Stauber and Pick in their book *Nutrition and Atherosclerosis* p.109, state:

> the ordinary bacon—eggs—buttered toast—creamed coffee breakfasts—with their huge intake of saturated fats, calories and cholesterol—should become the exception not the rule. They should be superseded by breakfasts made up of fruits, wholegrain cereals, skimmed milk . . . and spreads of honey, jam and marmalade used in moderation on whole grain breads.[45]

These three authors are some of the foremost research workers in the field of atherosclerosis in America. Their names are well known. Their recommendations could well be followed from the point of view of good general nutrition.

Foods containing a high proportion of cholesterol and hard fat are eggs, milk, cheese, butter, meat, fried foods, cream and pastries. Animal fats, or hard fats consist for the most part of palmitic and stearic acids and esters of these acids. Vegetable fats contain linoleic, oleic and arachidonic acids, which are unsaturated. A particular constituent of butter, myristic acid, has been shown to have potent cholesterol raising effect. In margarine the chemist has partially hardened the vegetable fat by hydrogenation, and the oil is often saturated. Normal margarine is of no use in lowering cholesterol, most brands having no effect either way on this blood component.[6]

In a recent survey of American diets,[8] of fats consumed, milk contributed 12%, butter 10%, hamburger steaks 9%, eggs 4%, margarine 4%, roast beef 4%, cream and vegetable shortening each 4%, ham, cheddar cheese, fruit pies, 'cookies' and ice cream all contributing 3% each item. The large contribution made by milk and butter fats to total fat consumption is seen in this analysis.

It has been the aim of modern research workers over the past years to prove their point by conducting clinical trials. Many such trials have been carried out to test whether coronary heart disease in a community can be controlled by lowering the intake of hard fat and cholesterol. It is difficult in such trials to control all the, variables sufficiently to satisfy statisticians and it is difficult often to ensure participants keep to a diet. Prospective trials show clearer results than retrospective as it would appear that once one has had a coronary it is difficult to modify prognosis by dietary measures. Christakis et al.[11] with the help of the anti-coronary club of New York subjected 814 men to a special low fat diet and reduced the incidence of coronary disease in these men. Their results were as follows:

Treated group: ...   3.39 cases/1,000 men
1st control group: ...   9.80 cases/1,000 men
2nd control group: ...   12.5 cases/1,000 men

The low fat diet for the treated group was made up of equal parts saturated, nonsaturated and polyunsaturated fatty acids. Three recent trials give good evidence of the protection afforded by a low animal fat diet. Turpeinen et al.[90] from Helsinki placed 327 men on a diet where soya bean oil replaced milk fat. Cholesterol level over a period of six years was lowered 51 mg below controls and triglycerides and phospholipids also lowered. Adipose tissue contained on analysis more linoleic and linolenic acid, and less myristic acid than controls. Electrocardiographs showed better results and coronary heart disease was of lower incidence. The trial ran for six years.

In post-infarction trials, Rinzler[82] and also Leren[52] show encouraging results in two recent trials. Rinzler put 941 men of the Acute Coronary Club of New York on a diet high in unsaturated fatty acids, and compared the health of the men over a number of years, to 457 males attending a cancer clinic who were eating normal diets. The heart patients on unsaturated fat diets had lower cholesterol and triglyceride levels and had an incidence of new coronary 'events' less than half that found amongst the control group. The prevalence of obesity and hypertension was also less in the treated group compared to controls. Leren from Oslo put 206 men between the ages of 30 and 64 years of age on a diet rich in vegetable oils (mainly soy bean oil) and low in animal fats and cholesterol. The men had all suffered a coronary attack. Their progress over a number of years was compared to controls who had similarly suffered a heart attack but who were not dieted. 27 sudden deaths were recorded in each group but whereas the vegetable fat group suffered 80 heart relapses, the control groups suffered 120. The differences were significant for those below the age of 60. Leren found that the blood cholesterol level had a far stronger relationship with incidence of coronary relapse than other treatable factors such as smoking, or blood pressure.

Geill and others (1962)[36] found that 133 patients over the age of 60 who took vegetable oils suffered four thrombotic episodes in ensuing years as against 15 amongst the control groups. Morrison in 1960,[71] treating 50 survivors from a myocardial infarct on a low fat intake of 25 gm/day, found that within 12 years the untreated group had all died whereas only 60% of the treated group had succumbed. Lyon and others in 1956[57] found that amongst post infarcted patients recurrence rate of heart disease could be reduced four times by the institution of a low fat diet. Negative results are reported by Rose (1965)[83] and Ball et al. (1965)[5] who found no benefit to result from treating patients with heart disease by special low fat diets, though these patients had already suffered a heart attack and therefore were less susceptible to improvement by dietary control.

The evidence is on the whole strong that overconsumption of hard fats plays a significant part in the aetiology of coronary heart disease.

Sugar

A certain school of research workers led by Professsor Yudkin champion sugar as the causal factor in coronary heart disease. As is often the case in rivalry within the laboratory or university, emotions run high on the matter, and tend to obscure the truth. The fat school wage war in the correspondence columns of learned journals against the sugar school, each trying to score points off the other, and in the process omitting and ignoring the more subtle complexities of this whole problem of aetiology. Let us examine the problem of sugar.

Until recently, a large consumption of carbohydrates and in particular sugar, was thought but a harmless and useful way of providing energy. Obesity was the only apparent danger and ten years ago at the end of a post war era obesity was seen as no real threat to life. However research has gathered momentum in ten years and is now pointing to various pathogenic and metabolic effects that follow upon the consumption and particularly the overconsumption of sucrose.

First of all an enormous increase in sugar consumption has occurred in the last 100 years,[67, 95] for there has been an eight fold increase in consumption since 1800 (see Fig. 9.1). Such a violent

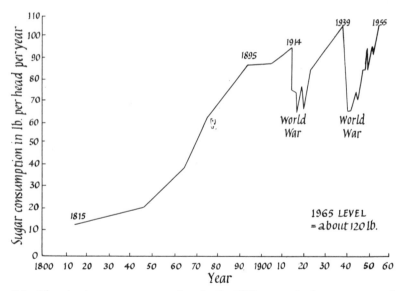

9.1 The rise in sugar consumption in the U.K. over the last century and a half (reproduced by kind permission of the authors from *Diabetes, Coronary Thrombosis, and the Saccharine Disease,* J. Wright, Bristol 1969)

shift in an environmental variable, and an important nutritional one, would seem to warrant some investigation as to the metabolic effects produced. These are now being undertaken by nutritionists.

Sucrose is replacing starch in our diet. In the first chapter in this book these changes are outlined in detail. Of carbohydrates in our diet, wheat, sugar and potatoes constitute 90%, and since 1880, wheat and potatoes have been cut by 50% in their consumption and sugar has risen 100% (Fig. 1.1). Total carbohydrate consumption has dropped from 490 to 408 gm.[42] Protein and fat consumption have risen. Sugar thus replaces bread and potatoes, and may soon provide as much calorie value as these two foodstuffs together. In the United States an even greater rise in consumption of sugar has taken place from a figure of 20 lb/head/year in 1845 to an estimated 130 lb/head/year at the present time. (Fig. 1.5).

Sucrose may play some part in the pathogenesis of atherosclerosis. Professor T. Tascher[88] for instance in Sofia fed chicks a sucrose rich diet over 16 weeks. The chicks showed higher blood lipid levels and more arteriosclerotic lesions than when fed a diet of glucose or cotton seed oil. Cholesterol levels also rose with the sucrose diet. Tascher places emphasis along with others on the fructose component of sucrose. Generally, sucrose has not been found to raise blood cholesterol levels , unless fed in large amounts.[51, 59] It has been found on the other hand to have a decisive effect upon serum triglyceride.[1, 51, 58] Cholesterol and triglyceride are metabolically inter-connected and it has been suggested that the serum triglycerides are more closely related to coronary artery disease than the blood cholesterol.[25, 50] Certainly they are raised in patients suffering an infarct. The metabolism of fat and carbohydrate in the body is interrelated at several points and the complexities of these relationships have yet to be fully worked out. The controversy over whether 'fat burns in the flame of carbohydrate' took place many years ago and livestock breeders know that carbohydrate can fatten animals. Interaction between sucrose and fat is referred to in the next section. It is sufficient to say here that sucrose adds to the high level of blood fats which provoke the formation of atheroma and prepare the ground for subsequent heart disease.

Apart from its metabolic effect upon blood fats and insulin. sucrose has the disadvantage nutritionally of providing only energy. As a food it contains no vitamins or minerals and as it satiates it has the propensity to *displace other more worthwhile foodstuffs from the diet.*

Professor Yudkin brought attention to bear upon this problem in connection with heart disease by his research reported in *The Lancet* of 1964.[94] Yudkin found that patients who had suffered a myocardial infarct had on analysis a higher intake of sucrose than controls. Similar findings were reported in those suffering from peripheral arterial disease. Dietary analysis, especially by recall or 24 hours' study, can be faulty and Yudkin's findings have been confirmed by some[72] and not by others.[54, 75] Osancova[72] is one of those who has confirmed Yudkin's findings. In Czechoslovakia for instance, a high epidemiological correlation has been found to exist between consumption of simple carbohydrates (sucrose) and death from heart disease, and in a more recent paper Osancova analyses the Ministry of Health records for that country and reveals that death rate from arteriosclerosis per 100,000 citizens varies more according to sucrose intake than fat intake. Death rate in areas of highest sucrose intake is 382 per 100,000 but 246 per 100,000 in the lowest consumption areas. Whilst with regard to fat consumption, in areas of high fat consumption death rate is 302 per 100,000 and 242 in low fat areas, a difference also though not so great a one.

Other strong support for Yudkin's thesis comes from the researches of A. M. Cohen and co-workers in Israel.[12] The evidence seems fairly convincing. A migration of Yemenites from Yemen to Israel has been taking place over a number of years in the Middle East. In the Yemen the people do not eat sugar. In Israel they do. In comparing men who had migrated recently to Israel with those who had immigrated a long time ago, far less diabetes and coronary thrombosis was found amongst the former group, the recent immigrants, than the latter. The cholesterol levels of the recent immigrants were also much lower. Dietary analysis to explain this showed no difference in fat consumption but a significant rise in sugar consumption in the older immigrants replacing consumption of bread. To confirm that sugar in place of bread could raise cholesterol levels in the blood, Groen et al.[34] in Israel interchanged bread and sucrose in the diet of volunteers and found that sucrose raised cholesterol readings in the volunteers by an amount which varied from 14.7 mg/100 ml to 27 mg. The glucose tolerance also worsened under the influence of sucrose feeding suggesting that this could possibly be the cause also of increased frequency of diabetes.[12]

However, in contrast, Papp et al.[75] and Little et al.[54] in dietary surveys amongst coronary patients found no evidence of an excessively high sucrose consumption in such patients, while Paul et al.[77] in a careful analysis of diets taken from a prospective trial under way in America found that coronary patients took more sugar but the significance of this was small. Cigarette consumption, coffee consumption, blood pressure level and cholesterol reading, with regard to the incidence of heart disease, showed greater statistical significance.

In a recent survey from Britain, Howell and Wilson[43] compared the sugar intake of 1,158 men believed free of ischemic heart disease with the intake of 170 men with confirmed or suspected heart disease. The diagnosis of heart disease was made by means of E.C.G. Difference in sugar consumption between the two groups was not found to be significant. People change their habits and the fact that a man has suspected heart disease may be enough to change eating habits considerably. Such pitfalls abound in this type of survey. However, whittling the number of subjects who had heart disease down to the 29 who had confirmed myocardial ischemia and who also had not changed their dietary habits over ten years Howell and Wilson still did not find significant differences in sucrose consumption though a small difference (580 g as compared to 510g) occurred between these smaller groups.

Studies of Burns Cox et al.[10] and of a Medical Research Council working party[66] were set up to test Yudkin's hypothesis, that sucrose was the factor responsible for coronary heart disease. Neither of these studies showed this. Burns Cox et al. concluded 'that the totality of data now available does not suggest that consumption of refined sugar is likely to be a major or specific factor in the production of myocardial infarction.' The Medical Research Council report concluded that 'the evidence in favour of a high sugar intake as a major factor in the development of myocardial infarction is extremely slender.'

From all this data it would appear that sucrose has yet to prove itself a dominant aetiological factor in coronary heart disease. Most of the evidence points to it being merely a contributory one. Factors such as consumption of animal fat, obesity and cigarette smoking have stronger evidence to suggest their significance in the causation of coronary heart disease.

171

The food and health of western man
Interaction of fat and sugar
In analysing present food trends in civilised communities rise in consumption of fat usually parallels rise in consumption of sugar. Yudkin[95] was the first to show this and pointed out how epidemiologically this fact could mislead nutritional workers. In terms of food eaten the two go often hand in hand and in such foods as pastries, cakes, puddings, chocolate, ice cream, are combined in the cooking and the preparation. It is not inconceivable that *both* play a pathogenic role in disease. It is highly probable that different components of the food we eat do interact upon one another, producing important metabolic results. Biochemistry is a long series of such interactions. R. R. McGandy and others[63] showed a potentiating effect on blood cholesterol when sucrose was added to a high fat diet and more particularly when sucrose and lactose were added to a high fat diet. (Don't add sugar to your Jersey cream!) Dumaswala and workers show that cane sugar potentiates hypercholesterolemia when given with coconut oil, and similarly nullifies the cholesterol lowering effect of safflower oil. M.A. Antar and co-workers[2] found that in lowering cholesterol the most effective combination was unsaturated fat in the diet *plus* low sugar. A. Keys and others[48] found similar interplay occurring between dietary carbohydrates and fat. Sucrose and coconut oil, (one of the few vegetable oils that is hard) raised the blood cholesterol to its highest level. Cereals with sunflower oil and potatoes and sunflower oil, on the other hand, were the combinations most effective in lowering cholesterol.

Obesity
Overnutrition, and the excess consumption of any food, be it protein, fat or carbohydrate produces obesity. The fact that sugar is available to more of us, and in such palatable profusion as afforded by modern food science, means that more of us eat for the sake of eating rather than because we are hungry. Calories are concentrated in sweetened and refined foods and 'fool the appetite'. Sucrose is by no means the only culprit in the promotion of excess body tissue though it is a potent factor. Refining of flour and the high consumption following of pastries, cakes, biscuits and such snacks contributes in very large measure to obesity.

In general, morbidity and mortality are higher amongst the overweight than amongst those whose weight is normal.[62] Obesity is correlated with high blood pressure[23] and also with high blood cholesterol.[23] Both these further factors predispose towards coronary heart disease. However obesity is common in the United States and many obese men escape having coronaries. Obesity is also correlated with many other diseases besides heart disease, as explained elsewhere in this book. It is therefore perhaps not surprising that in some early studies overweight did not figure strongly as a mortality factor in heart disease, though definitely affecting prognosis to an extent. Obesity per se is probably a less potent risk factor than raised serum cholesterol or high blood pressure. In the Framingham study, overweight appeared to increase the cardiac workload and in those with compromised coronary circulation brought on angina or predisposed to sudden death. Independent of blood pressure or lipid abnormalities the obese were prone to sudden death where others were not.

The frugal diet

If obesity follows from modern dietary standards and modern social patterns, then the study of a way of life that lies at the opposite extreme to this, where dietary intake is frugal and social life uncomplicated and unhurried, should reveal some interesting comparisons. Studies have been made in this respect of religious communities and groups eating special diets. Rice diets, vegetarian and fruitarian diets have all been used in the study of heart disease and provide some interesting material for commentary.

In Belgium, J. J. Groen and others[32] examined the health and food of Trappist monks and compared this group to Benedictine monks. The Trappists had the more frugal diet, eating a breakfast of brown bread (78% extraction), a lunch of potatoes, vegetables and a little margarine, porridge and fresh fruit and an evening meal of peas and beans, brown bread and cheese: a vegetarian diet. The Benedictines on the other hand ate meat, butter, eggs, fish and sugar. The Trappists had a very much lower level of cholesterol than the Benedictines, though both groups had a low incidence of heart disease compared to the outside world. This low overall incidence was thought due to the calm contemplative life led by the monks. The beneficial effect of this way of life was thought to overrule any dietary indiscretion. It was however pointed out that the Trappists' diet won on points by producing a lower cholesterol level!

W. Kempner in 1948[46] reported a series of significant experiments where patients severely ill with hypertensive vascular disease were put on a 2,000 calorie diet consisting of rice, sugar, fruit and unsweetened fruit juices; a simple diet and in fact rather monotonous diet. The sugar consumed was 100 gm a day, about half our average consumption today. Kempner lowered the blood cholesterol by this means from 273 to 177 mg in his patients and found that 75% of his severely ill patients made marked clinical improvement, without medication or treatment with drugs such as Digitalis. It seems on the whole remarkable that these experiments have been largely overlooked. The monotony of the diet may have contributed to lack of enthusiasm. They are well written up however in Kempner's original paper with good clinical evidence relating to the cases and would seem to justify further research. Restricted protein, carbohydrates· and fat, with the allowance of plenty of raw fruit and fruit juices is by and large the diet recommended by the naturopath. though no doubt the sugar would be frowned upon! The diet provided a large potassium intake which seemed in no way to disturb Kempner's patients, their serum levels of potassium remaining constant, their urine excretion only increasing. The very low sodium and chloride levels in the food enabled cases of oedema resistant to mercurial diuretics to respond well to the regime. 140 patients were treated, and clinical improvement was noted in size of heart, E.C.G. findings, eyegrounds and blood pressure. In no instance was there deterioration in clinical condition. An analysis of this rice-fruit diet revealed a breakdown as follows: 2,000 calories, 20 g protein, 5 g fat, 700-1,000 cc fruit juice, supplementary vitamins, A, D, and B, and 100 g sugar. The diet contained approximately 200 mg chloride and 150 mg sodium. Its benefits strongly derived from the low fat and low sodium content.

It might be mentioned in passing that some of the poorer parts of the world exist mainly on rice and vegetables and rice may provide up to 85% of the total calories eaten in Asian countries. Surprisingly good health can be maintained on such a diet. The level of the blood fats (the triglycerides and cholesterol) in these peoples is very low and heart disease uncommon.

Recently C. Watanakunakorn[91] confirmed Kempner's findings on two patients, both with poorly controlled diabetes and numerous eyeground changes with exudates and haemorrhages. Cholesterol was lowered in both on the rice diet, in one case from 212 mg to

174

162 mg and in the other from 300 mg to 173 mg. Vision was generally improved and in one case the insulin requirement also dropped significantly.

Vitamin C

Vitamin C and the consumption of vegetables and fruit definitely affects serum cholesterol levels, and almost certainly the production of atheroma. Vitamin C is essential for the laying down of the arterial ground substance.[92, 93] It reduces triglycerides in the blood[85] and lowers the level of ß lipoproteins. If vitamin C levels are low, blood fats tend to rise. High doses of ascorbic acid on the other hand reduce the cholesterol concentration in blood.[28, 85]

Pectin is a carbohydrate found in the skin and rind of citrus fruit, apples, vegetables and sunflower seeds. It composes 0.2% to 1% of the fruit. Oral pectin has been shown to increase faecal cholesterol and lower serum cholesterol showing another useful quality appertaining to fruits and vegetables.[26, 53, 74]

The vegetarian diet

The Trappist monks, previously mentioned, lived on a vegetarian diet. Their cholesterol level was noted as much lower than the Benedictines. Vegetable protein in the form of legumes[56] and again rice and oats[17] has been shown to lower cholesterol. In an interesting comparison between the diet of an Italian labourer and that of an American labourer A. Keys and others[48] have shown that the Italian had a healthier cholesterol level. His diet contained more fruit, legumes and cereals and less of the so-called 'rich' foods— milk, meat and sugar, that the American consumed.

In another study Grande and others[30] showed that beans, lima beans, and split peas were cholesterol lowering foods as compared to soy beans and sugar. Hodges and others,[41] Groen et al.,[31] and Kinsell and co-workers[49] have all showed that vegetarian protein diets lower cholesterol.

Smoking

A relationship between smoking and coronary heart disease had been suspected on clinical grounds for many years. Mortality data[35] and field studies[19, 86] have confirmed this suspicion. American data from Framingham[19] has shown that heavy cigarette smokers have a five fold increased rate of sudden death from coronary

175

disease as compared to their non-smoking counterparts. The risk could be normalised by the giving up of smoking. The Surgeon-General's Advisory Committee in the U.S.A. in an analysis of 26,000 deaths also point to the increased mortality from heart disease that is associated with smoking.[81] Incidence of heart disease is directly proportional also to the number of cigarettes smoked.[18] If the cholesterol count is raised and the blood pressure is high; smoking will kill with fair certainty.

Exercise

An ingenious study of London bus drivers and their conductors, showed that the drivers were more likely to die from sudden coronary thrombosis than the conductors.[68] Another study showed that government clerks suffered more often from fatal heart disease than postmen.[68] From this and other studies it was suggested that a relationship existed between physical activity and the incidence of ischemic heart disease. In a study of 5,000 post mortem examinations, of men between 45 and 70, Morris and Crawford conclude also that physical activity gives protection against coronary heart disease,[69] and find that myocardial infarct, and the actual thrombosis itself is protected against more than the atherosclerosis or state of the arterial vessel. Exercise may encourage a better collateral circulation, prevent coagulation in the blood or contribute by lowering serum lipids.

Psychological stress

Reference has been made to the difficulty of measuring this factor, and studies are therefore few and often inconclusive in this field. However in one trial[84] of 100 men between the ages of 25 and 40, who had suffered from heart disease, in comparing these men to 100 controls, it was found that of the heart patients 91 gave a. history of severe occupational strain which was found in only 20 of the controls. The type of stress encountered was often severe and was concerned with internal tension, as opposed to the external stress of 'flood, pestilence and war'! L. E. Hinkle and others[39] found in America that executives who rose through the ranks had higher rates of coronary disease than executives who were not so successful. One fears executives in Britain might have a lower incidence of heart disease than their American colleagues!

These findings are confirmed by those reported from the Du

Pont Company in America where executives had half the incidence of myocardial infarction of men in the lowest salary class who were aiming to better their position.[79] Differences in cholesterol, blood pressure, smoking and weight could not explain away this difference.

Differences in personality have been noted between coronary patients and non-coronary patients[24] but such factors may be merely associative and not causal. Working long hours has been found to be related to excessive mortality from coronary disease[9] (as also related to peptic ulcer) though a retrospective study by Bainton and Peterson[3] did not reveal that excessive 'drive' at work was so associated. These factors are however difficult to measure, and require further study.

Prevalence
Coronary heart disease is the disease of our time. It is said that there is an epidemic of this condition in the West. Four out of 10 men will die from the disease and two out of 10 women. What is more alarming than this is the manner in which younger and younger men are succumbing to the illness. Fig. 9.2 and Table 9.1 show the nature of this increase. In the younger group between the ages of 45 and 64 the incidence of heart disease has *almost doubled in* 17 *years.*

Post mortem records are more accurate than death certificates for assessing cause of death. Analysis of the post mortem records at the London Hospital[70, 76] showed a *sevenfold* increase in 40 years in the number of cases of coronary heart disease found in persons dying between the ages of 35 and 70. In England and Wales during the course of a year nearly half a million persons are diagnosed as suffering from ischemic heart disease.[89] Approximately 100,000 in the course of a year will die from this disease. The increase, as already stated, has been greatest in the middle age group. In a recent study by Reid et al.[80] almost 12% of men between the ages of 50 and 59 in Britain showed evidence of heart disease. The evidence in this case was from electrocardiographic analysis. The same workers recorded a 21% frequency of disease in Americans of the same age. The increased severity of the disease in the States was thought due to the greater incidence of obesity.

The distressing aspect of this problem is that heart disease is now a young man's disease. It is now routine on the part of a

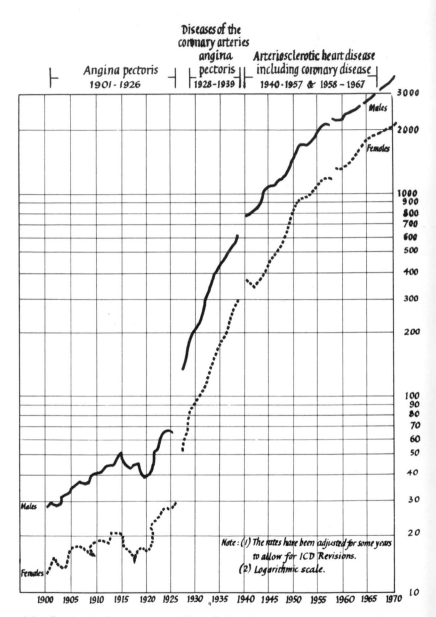

9.2 Crude death rate per million living from angina pectoris; diseases of the coronary arteries, angina pectoris; arteriosclerotic heart disease including coronary disease, England and Wales, 1901-1970 (from Registrar General's Statistical Review of England and Wales, various years)

pathologist to expect to find atheroma in a young man's arteries. Of United States soldiers killed in action 15% of the men were found to have plaques of atheroma in the coronary arteries, occluding half or more of the lumen.[21] In another study, in New Orleans,[87] the prevalence of coronary fibrous plaques was 17% in males (white) between the ages of 10 and 19, while 45% of those examined between the ages of 20 and 29 had such plaques in the coronary arteries. In 1963 40% of British males who died from this disease

TABLE 9.1
Mortality from coronary heart disease in
males and females aged between 45 and 64 years.

Year	Males	Females
	Death rate per million living	
1953	2712	731
1958	3457	876
1963	4333	1049
1970	4822	1255

Source: Registrar General's Statistical Reviews.
Table 17a. Categories 410-414

were under 65. Women are less prone till later in life. All these findings are similarly reported from other countries where industrialisation and civilisation have advanced at a fast rate. Highest death rates for coronary thrombosis are found in South Africa, England, Scotland, U.S.A. and Scandinavia.

It is interesting in the study of the history of this disease to find that one is dealing with a condition that was indeed rare 50 years ago. L. Michaels[67] in an interesting historical survey of heart disease has found one description of angina (heart pain) in Graeco-Roman times, none in Mediaeval and Renaissance periods and one in the seventeenth century (the Earl of Clarendon's angina). Heberden in 1802,[38] one of the great physicians of the past, described angina as a condition which 'hardly had a place . . . in medical books'. Gout and Migraine are both well documented down the ages. Angina though is conspicuous by its absence. Balfour in

1876[4] saw only two cases in his time at the Edinburgh Royal Infirmary and Osler in 1910[73] had not seen a single patient before becoming a Fellow of the Royal College of Physicians in the United States. Paul White, a famous heart physician saw his *first* case of Ischemic Heart Disease causing angina in 1921 in his second year of private practice. These are facts which are hard for us to accept nowadays when heart disease is such a universal malady and the topic has become so commonplace. Nevertheless, the facts of history are as recorded, and the figures of today speak for themselves.

Summary

The author is biased in favour of a nutritional cause for coronary heart disease and a nutritional solution! However this is not to ignore the evidence that smoking, stress and lack of exercise also play a significant part. In fact heart disease is the direct result of our western civilised way of living. The diet is too rich and refined, and we lack the open air, exercise and a more natural way of living that is excluded from the environment of our big cities.

Could heart disease be prevented? In large measure, yes. The ideal diet would be low or absent in sugar, low in refined carbohydrates, low in animal fat and high in vegetables and fruit. It need not necessarily be frugal but should avoid heavy meats (beef, mutton) and meals should be light. In other words the evidence here presented favours the 'McCarrison diet' (see Chapter 14), a diet based on wholegrain cereals, fruit and vegetable and light meat. A simple solution and not at all impractical but unlikely to be taken up by the majority of people. Habits and food habits particularly die hard, and until the evidence is overwhelming the majority are unlikely to be moved.

REFERENCES TO CHAPTER 9

1 Anderson J. T., Grande F., Matsumoto Y., Keys A., *J. Nutr.* 1963, 79:349.
2 Antar M. A., Ohlson M. A., Hodges R. E., *Amer. J. Clin. Nutr.* 1964, 14:169.
3 Bainton C. R., Peterson D. R., *New Eng. J. Med.* 1963, 268:569.
4 Balfour G. W. *Clinical lectures on diseases of Heart and Aorta*, J. A. Churchill, London 1876.
5 Ball K. P., Harrington E., McAllen P. M., Pilkington T. R. E., Richards J. M., Sowry G., *The Lancet* 1965, 2:501.

6 Beveridge J. M. R., Connell W. F., *Amer. J. Clin. Nutr.* 1962, 10:391.
7 *Brit. Med. J.* 1971, 4:64.
8 Browe J., Morley D. M., Logrillo V., Doyle J., *J. Amer. Diet Ass.* 1967, 50:376.
9 Buell P., Breslow L., *J. Chron. Dis.* 1960, 11:615.
10 Burns Cox C. J., Doll R., Ball K. P., *Brit. Heart J.* 1969, 31:485.
11 Christakis G. J., Rinzler S. H., Archer M. S., Jampel S., *Amer. J. Publ. Hlth.* 1966, 56:299.
12 Cohen A. M., Teitelbaum A., Balogh M., Groen J. J., *Amer. J. Clin. Nutr.* 1966, 19:59.
13 Crawford M. A. *The Lancet* 1969, 2:1419, *The Lancet* 1968, 1:1329.
14 Crawford M. D., Gardner M. J., Morris J. N., *The Lancet* 1971, 2:327.
15 Dawber T. R., Moore F. E., Mann G. V. *Amer. J. Publ. Hlth.* 1957, 47.4.
16 ——, Kannel W. B., Revotskie N., Kagan A., *Proc. Roy. Soc. Med.* 1962, 55:265.
17 De Groot A. P., Lukyen R., Pikaer N. *The Lancet* 1963, 2:303.
18 Doll W. R., Hill A. B., *Brit. Med. J.* 1964 1:1399.
19 Doyle J. T., Dawber T. R., Kannel W. B., Heslin A. S., Kahn H. A., *J. Amer. Med. Ass.* 1964, 190:886.
20 Dumaswala V. J., Modak A. J., Divakaran P., *The Lancet* 1970, 2:724
21 Enos W. F., Beyer J. C., Holmes R. H., *J. Amer. Med. Ass.* 1955, 158:912.
22 Epstein F. H., *J. Chron. Dis.* 1965, 18:735.
23 ——, Francis T., Haynes N. H., Johnson B. C., *Amer. J. Epidemiol.* 1965, 81:307.
24 ——, in *Modern Trends in Cardiology* ed. A. Morgan Jones, Butterworth, London 1960.
25 Farrehi C., Perley A., Ritzmann L. W., Malinow L. R., *Circulation* 1968, 38: Suppl. 6, p.6.
26 Fisher D. H., *Med. World News,* May 14, 1965, 6:86.
27 Friedman M., Rosenman R. H., Carroll V., *Circulation* 1958, 17:852.
28 Ginter E., Bobek P., Babala J., *Cor. Vasa* 1969, 11:65.
29 Gordon T., Kannel B. *The Community as an Epidemiological Laboratory* ed. I. Kessler, M. L. Levin, John Hopkins Press, Baltimore, 1970, p.123.
30 Grande F., Anderson J. T., Keys A., *J. Nutr.* 1965, 86:313.
31 Groen J. J., Tijong B. K., Kaminga C., Willebrands A., *Voeding* 1952, 13:556.
32 ——, Tijong K., Koster M., Willebrands A., Verdonck G., Pierloot M., *Amer. J. Clin. Nutr.* 1962, 10:456.
33 ——, Balogh M., Yaron E., Freeman J., *Amer. J. Clin. Nutr.* 1965, 17:296.
34 ——, ——, ——, Cohen A. M., *Amer. J. Clin. Nutr.* 1966, 19:46.
35 Hammond E. C., Horn D., *J. Amer. Med. Ass.* 1958, 166:1159.
36 Hansen P. F., Geill T., Lund E., *The Lancet* 1962, 2:1193.
37 Hatch F. T., Reissell P., Poon-King T. M. W., Canellos G., *Circulation* 1966, 33:679.
38 Herberden W. *Commentary on the History and Cure of Diseases* 1802, Reprinted N.Y. Acad. Med. The History of Med. Series 18.
39 Hinkle L. E., Whitney L. H., Lehman E. *Confer. on Cardiovasc. Dis. Amer. Ht. Ass. Chicago* 1, 2:64.

40 Hodges R. E., Krehl W. A., *Amer. J. Clin. Nutr.* 1965, 17:334.
41 ——, ——, Stone, D., Lopez A., *Amer. J. Clin. Nutr.* 1967, 20:198.
42 Hollingsworth D. F., Greaves J. P., *Amer. J. Clin. Nutr.* 1967, 20:65.
43 Howell R. W., Wilson D. G., *Brit. Med. J.* 1969, 3:145.
44 Hubbard A. W., Pocklington W. D., *J. Sci. Fd. Agric.* 1968, 19:571.
45 Katz L. N., Stamler J., Pick R., *Nutrition and Atherosclerosis* 1959, H. Kimpton.
46 Kemper W., *Amer. J. Med.* 1948, 4:445.
47 Keys A., *J. Amer. Med. Ass.* 1957, 164:1912.
48 ——, Anderson J. T., Grande F., *J. Nutr.* 1960, 70:257.
49 Kinsell L. W., Partridge J., Boling L., Margen S., *J. Clin. Endocrin* 1952, 12:909.
50 Kuo P. T., *J. Amer. Med. Ass.* 1967, 201:101.
51 ——, Bassett D. R., *Ann. Int. Med.* 1965, 62:1199.
52 Leren P., *Bull N.Y. Acad. Med.* 1968, 44:1012.
53 Leveille G. A., Sauberlich H. E., *J. Nutr.* 1966, 88:209.
54 Little J. A., Shanoff H. M., Czima A., Yano R., *The Lancet* 1966, 1:732.
55 Lowenstein F. W., *Amer. J. Clin. Nutr.* 1964, 15:175.
56 Lukyen R., Pikaer N., Polman H., Schippers F., *Voeding*, 1962, 23:447.
57 Lyon T. P., Yeakley A., Gofman J. W., Strusower B., *Calif. Med.* 1956, 84:325.
58 Macdonald I., Braithwaite D. M., *Clin. Sci.* 1964, 27:23.
59 ——, *Wld. Rev. Nutr. Diet* 1967, 8:143.
60 Malmros H., *The Lancet* 1969, 2:479.
61 Marks H. H., *Metabolism* 1957, 6:417.
62 ——, *Bull N.Y. Acad. Med.* 1960, 36:296.
63 McGandy R. B., Hegsted D. M., Myers M. L., Stare F. J., *Amer. J. Clin. Nutr.* 1966, 18:237.
64 *Med. Jour. Austral.* 1967, 1:309.
65 *Medical News Tribune*, Aug. 27, 1971, vol. 3, No. 35.
66 Medical Research Council Working Party, *The Lancet* 1970, 2:1265.
67 Michaels L., *Brit. Ht. J.* 1966, 28:258.
68 Morris J. N., Heady J. A., Raffle P., Roberts C. G., Parks J. W., *The Lancet* 1953, 2:1053.
69 Morris J. N., Crawford M. D., *Brit. Med. J.* 1958, 2:1485.
70 Morris J. N., *The Lancet* 1951, 1:1 and 69.
71 Morrison L. M., *J. Amer. Med. Ass.* 1960, 173:884.
72 Osancova K., Hejda S., Zvolankova K., *The Lancet* 1965, 1:494.
73 Osler W., *Modern Medicine*, vol. 1. Lea., Philadelphia and New York, 1907.
74 Palmer G. H., Dixon D. G., *Amer. J. Clin. Nutr.* 1966, 18:437.
75 Papp O. A., Padilla L., Johnson A. L., *The Lancet* 1965, 2:259.
76 Parish H. M., *J. Chron. Dis.* 1961, 14:326.
77 Paul O., MacMillan A., McKean H., Park H., *The Lancet* 1968, 2:1049.
78 ——, Lepper, M. H., Phelan W. H., Dupertuis G., Macmillan A., *Circulation* 1963, 28:20.
79 Pell S., D'Alonzo C. A., *J. Occp. Med.* 1961, 3:467.
80 Reid D. D., Holland W. W., Rose G. A., *The Lancet* 1967, 2:1375.
81 *Report of the Advisory Committee of the Surg. Genl. of Publ. Health Serv. Publ. Health Serv.*, Publ. No. 1103. U.S. Govt. Printing Office, Washington D.C. 1964.
82 Rinzler S. H., *Bull, N.Y. Acad. Med.* 1968, 44:936.

83 Rose G. A., Thompson W. B., Williams R. T., *Brit Med. J.* 1965, 1:1531.
84 Russek H. I., Zohman B. L., *Amer. J. Med. Sci.* 1958, 235:266.
85 Sokoloff B., Hori M., Saelhof C. C., Wrzolek T., *J. Amer. Ger. Soc.* 1966, 14:1239.
86 Spain D. M., Nathan D. J., *J. Amer. Med. Ass.* 1961, 177:683.
87 Strong J. P., McGill H. C., *Amer. J. Path.* 1962, 40:37.
88 Tascher T., *Internat. Med. Trib. G.B.,* Oct. 5, 1967, p.11.
89 *The Common Illness of our Time.* Office of Health Economics, 1966, p.18.
90 Turpeinen O., Miettinen M., Karvonen M. J., Roine P., Pekkarinen M., Lehtosno E. J., *Amer. J. Clin. Nutr.* 1968, 21:255.
91 Watanakunakorn C., *Med. Wld. News,* May 14, 1965, p.84.
92 Willis G. C., *Can. Med. Ass. J.* 1953, 69:17.
93 ——, Tishman S., *Can. Med. Ass. J.* 1955, 72:500.
94 Yudkin J., *The Lancet* 1964, 2:4.
95 ——, *Proc. Nutr. Soc.* (Lond.) 1964, 23:2:149.
96 ——,Moreland J., *The Lancet* 1966, 2:1359.

183

Ten

Refined carbohydrates and disease: 'The Cleave Hypothesis'

The theory is simple, deceptively so. It might even appear to some to be too simple for acceptance, that refined carbohydrates cause disease. The 'Cleave hypothesis' is best studied in Cleave's own book *Diabetes, Coronary Thrombosis and the Saccharine Disease* by T. L. Cleave and G. D. Campbell.[26] It is well worth reading and the arguments are presented lucidly and logically. All doctors, nutritionists and interested persons should read it as in this book lie clues to the causation of much degenerative disease prevalent in the Western world today.

The principal argument propounded can be summarised as follows. During the last hundred years there has been a radical change wrought in western man's diet. His food has become sweet and refined. That is to say, carbohydrates which provide the foundation of man's diet, his main source of calories, have been subject to processing. Flour is now refined to 70% extraction, and sugar an excessively refined food is consumed in abundance as pure sucrose. As a consequence the fibre in the diet has been depleted and human intestinal function suffers as a consequence. Excess consumption of refined carbohydrate leads to such diseases as peptic ulcer, diverticulitis, haemorrhoids, cancer of the colon and varicose veins. Furthermore the upset in colonic microflora brought about by this diet leads to cholecystitis, appendicitis and pyelonephritis whereas the metabolic stress upon the body produces obesity, diabetes and coronary heart disease! Dental caries and periodontal disease merely add to the score!

The universality and importance of such a unitary theory of disease tends either to impress one or turn one away. The fashion nowadays is to look for multi-factorial aetiology, to number many

184

Refined carbohydrates and disease
factors that contribute to chronic disease and propose that the complexity of aetiology is too difficult to unravel, chronic disease too complex to prevent. It would seem to the author that the truth of the matter lies between the two. There are obviously dominant factors in aetiology and minor factors. The dominant factor in obesity is obviously over-consumption of sweetened refined food and a minor factor is lack of exercise. The dominant factor in aetiology of dental caries and periodontal disease is the consumption of sweet sticky carbohydrates and a minor factor certain trace element deficiencies. Cleave has brought together in his book epidemiological evidence to incriminate the consumption of refined carbohydrate in many diseases and names it as the dominant factor in each case. One would dispute as to whether the dominance is truly present in every case, but the general thesis is sound.

In contrast to the approach taken up by Cleave and Campbell in their book on the Saccharine Disease, it has been the intention of the author, in this present work, to emphasise how the modern-day diet is deficient in *several* characteristics, *one* of these being the high consumption of refined carbohydrates. For it has definitely been shown for instance that high consumption of animal fats is contributory to heart disease. The deficiency too of vegetables and fruit in the diet is seen as contributory to poor health generally, and deficiency of minerals and trace elements has been highlighted where appropriate as leading to ill-health. All of these factors should be considered in any treatise dealing with nutrition and disease and not one factor in isolation.

Most of all it is necessary to consider the place of psychological stress in causation of disease. To ignore psychology is to ignore the most important factor of all. A healthy mind forms a healthy body. A sick mind, unhappiness, discontent, or anxiety lead to bodily ill-health. Psychosomatic medicine is a huge problem contemporarily and to sweep it all aside as such enthusiasts as Cleave and Campbell are wont to do, as irrelevant, is shortsighted and self-defeating. The total environment and its effect upon total man is in the final analysis the proper subject of study.

Epidemiological arguments
Cleave in his book bases much of his deductions upon the data of epidemiological research. He contrasts prevalence of

185

certain diseases in India and Africa with prevalence in countries of western civilisation, and shows how much more common these conditions are in the west. He reinforces his argument particularly by showing how Africans in America suffer these diseases of civilisation but Africans in native Africa are free from them. He also shows how the Indians that settled in Natal, South Africa, took on the same degenerative diseases white men suffered from but were free from these at home. This result of urbanisation he attributes to the overconsumption of white flour and sugar. This particular change of nutrition could certainly be a factor of importance but one must remember that many other nutritional factors are subtly altered in the process of western urbanisation as well. Social habits and customs undergo drastic reshaping and such factors as lack of exercise, smoking, and psychological stresses also play a significant part in aetiology. To stress but one factor in urbanisation as relevant to disease aetiology even though this factor may be a dominant one, is not wise. However, Cleave and Campbell wrote their book to make a certain point and the impact of such a book rests upon clarity and strength in the presentation and it may seem unimportant to quibble over minor differences.

An eminent authority in the epidemiological field, Denis Burkitt (of Burkitt's lymphoma) has recently lent his weight to Cleave and Campbell in the establishment of their new hypothesis. Burkitt has outlined in several papers[17, 18] the rightness of epidemiological thinking put forward by Cleave and Campbell and agrees largely with their ideas concerning aetiology. He has also added a further disease to Cleave's list for consideration, namely cancer of the colon, putting forward suggestive evidence that this is caused by a diet high in refined carbohydrate. Burkitt has high regard for the work of Cleave.

The stress of simple carbohydrates

Important metabolic differences are now found to exist between starch and sucrose with regard to their physiological reactions within the human body.[65] Much of this difference of action stems from varying absorption rate. Sucrose is absorbed several times faster than starch due to its simpler structure. As a consequence, a more rapid rise of blood sugar levels follows sucrose ingestion.[28, 96] This rise in blood sugar is followed by a rapid rise in blood insulin[97] and a later rise in blood triglyceride levels.[5, 58, 65]

Every deviation from the homeostatic norm within the body has if possible to be countered and resolved by means of body physiological mechanisms. The greater rise in blood sugar levels following the ingestion of sucrose as compared to starch means greater stress is laid upon these physiological mechanisms to restore the homeostatic norm.

It is not considered necessary here to detail how this restoration is carried out or upon what factors it depends. Research work in the field of carbohydrate physiology is fast unfolding, with regard to sucrose, fat and insulin biochemistry. The data is accumulating day by day on the mechanisms that control the interactions of these three substances and the field is a complex one.[95] It is sufficient to say that a certain amount of evidence exists to show that the pathogenesis of obesity[81, 101] disorders of insulin (over and under production) [31, 49, 96] diabetes[3, 13, 37] and atherosclerosis[29, 80, 99] are closely linked to the handling of body sugars.

Ingestion of starch and protein seems to be taken more quietly by the body than ingestion of sucrose.[28, 96] Blood sugar homeostasis is disturbed less by these more complex foodstuffs. Output of human growth hormone and adrenalin is affected by even a small deviation of blood sugar level. A rise or fall of 10 mg/100 ml blood sugar can affect output of these homones[64] and blood pressure readings at different times of the day have also been shown to relate to blood sugar levels. Large deviations in blood sugar levels brought about by the ingestion of sucrose are therefore to be discouraged.

Cheraskin and Ringsdorf[24] in an interesting experiment fed volunteers a high protein low sucrose diet and reduced the blood pressure variation throughout the day as a result of this. The blood sugar levels varied less. Rats and humans fed on diets rich in complex carbohydrates and protein also produce, on oral glucose tolerance testing, a smaller variation in blood sugar.[27, 98] Rats (and humans) fed sucrose diets on the other hand show diabetic abnormality after a certain period.[27, 98] Sucrose ingestion can thus stress insulin regulating mechanisms.

Functional hypoglycemia is becoming now more commonly diagnosed[92] and may follow ingestion of sucrose rich meals. The symptoms of this complaint are the symptoms of hypoglycemia and include pallor, sweating, nervousness, tremor and hunger. The condition may be a prelude to diabetes in that poor control of

187

insulin release within the body is thought to be present in the condition.[71, 87] A glucose tolerance test often reveals a rapid rise of blood sugar followed by a long fall leading to hypoglycemia. Insulin release, late and poorly regulated, is thought to be the cause of the hypoglycemia, which occurs commonly 2 to 3 hours after eating. Frequent or excessive sucrose feeding could contribute to such an abnormal state.

Claude Bernard[35] emphasised the need for homeostasis. He stated that at all levels of biological organisation in plants as well as in animals, survival and fitness are conditioned by the ability of the organism to resist the impact of the outside world and maintain constant, within narrow limits, the physiochemical characteristics of the internal environment. The ingestion of much sucrose throws a strain upon the organism that can upset the homeostatic mechanisms that govern the complicated metabolic relationships within the body. The ingestion of much sucrose is therefore on evidence a course not to be highly recommended.

Analysis of aetiology

The chronic diseases specified by Cleave, Campbell, Painter and Burkitt as those that develop following consumption of refined carbohydrate will be shortly reviewed in this and following chapters. The full list of associated diseases is as follows:

Coronary thrombosis
Obesity
Diabetes
Peptic ulcer
Diverticulitis
Varicose veins
Haemorrhoids
Dental caries
Periodontal disease
Cancer of the colon
Pyelonephritis
Cholecystitis
Appendicitis
Renal stones.

The first four specified here have been reviewed in separate chapters. A short summary on each of the other conditions mentioned follows. It is also important to note here that association occurs geographically between this group of diseases and within the same individual, suggesting common aetiology.[18, 78, 79]

Diverticulitis

This disease called once the 'appendicitis of the colon' occurs in the elderly and presents with abdominal pain and obstruction of the sigmoid colon in the left iliac fossa. On examination of the inflamed bowel multiple small sacs, called diverticulae, are seen protruding through a thickened, inflamed and oedematous bowel wall, the lumen of which is narrowed. It is supposed that the diverticulae are herniations of the mucus membrane through the colonic wall, forced out through colonic pressure, later becoming inflamed as a result of faecal impaction.

N. S. Painter[75, 76, 77] has recently carried out a series of experiments on the human colon to estimate pressures within the lumen when contraction is taking place both in healthy subjects and those with diverticulosis. Contraction was seen to occur within the colon by a process of segmentation; this process forcing the bowel contents onwards. Segmentation occurred spontaneously or as a result of emotion, mechanical stimuli or drugs (morphine). Animal experiments show that a refined diet narrows the colon, a bulky diet enlarges it. It is postulated that a refined diet produces a viscous non-bulky stool. To effectively propel this viscous mass, the colon has to narrow down, producing excessive segmentation and increased pressure. Under these conditions the herniation of diverticulae takes place and further constipation brings about inflammation of this disintegrated bowel wall.

Painter and Burkitt[78] marshal evidence and argument to show how this disease originates from the chronic consumption of a *low fibre diet*. The dramatic rise in incidence of diverticulosis has occurred only in economically developed countries. The transit times of bowel contents in these countries is much slower than in undeveloped countries where the disease is rare (Fig. 10.1). The bulk of the faeces is much larger in native Africans than in this country. (Fig. 10.2). The low residue diet in this country is due to high consumption of sugar and refined flour replacing unrefined. It is also due to the palatability and ease of consumption of *all* processed foods.

Carlson and Hoelzel[23] by feeding a number of diets varying

189

in fibre and cellulose content showed that refined diets in rats narrowed the colon and led to the formation of diverticulae, while bulky diets rich in cellulose prevented this. Morgan and Ellis[72] recently repeated the experiment over a shorter time period and producd narrow colons in rats.

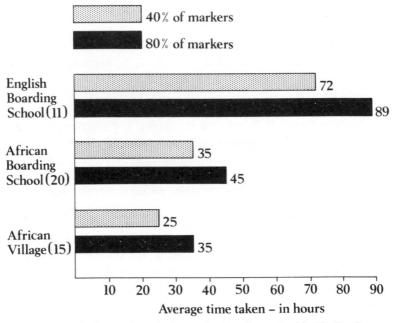

10.1 Effect of diet on intestinal transit time (from Burkitt D. P., *Cancer*, 1971, 28:3)

Kyle et al.[59] and Cleave and Campbell[26] in their book emphasise the difference in prevalence of this disease between civilised and uncivilised peoples. Kyle et al. found a thirty to forty fold difference between Europeans and natives living in Singapore and Fiji and an even greater difference when native incidence of the disease was compared to incidence of the disease in Scotland (Table 10.1). Racial factors, ease of diagnosis, availability of medical diagnosis, average age of population could all account for a greater frequency of diverticulitis in countries such as England and Scotland as compared to Fiji or Hong Kong. Racial studies

190

show that when natives from one region emigrate to an urbanised region their frequency of disease increases.

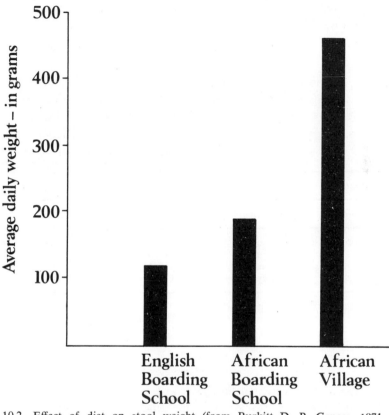

10.2 Effect of diet on stool weight (from Burkitt D. P. *Cancer,* 1971, 28 : 3)

    Rural Africans such as the Zulu eat a bulky diet of unrefined maize and vegetables. They have a low incidence of diverticulitis. At the Charles Johnson Memorial Hospital in Natal no case of diverticulitis has been recorded in the rural African.[26] Yet when the African takes to the town and to civilised ways of living his diverticulitis rate goes up. The negro in the United States now has a frequency rate with regard to this disease which is as high as his white compatriot, soft food of western society contributing to this.

The softer diet leads to a more viscous stool and a slower passage through the intestines. The African has a bowel motion twice a day, the Englishman once a day.[33] Barium meal studies confirm that transit time of food through the intestine is twice as fast in the African as the Englishman.[21]

TABLE 10.1

Number of cases admitted and annual admission rates for colonic diverticulitis in the various ethnic groups in four different countries studied

Country	Type of Population	Population Served	No. of cases	Prevalence of diverticulitis per annum per 100,000 population	Av. age
1. Scotland	European	400,000	206	12.88	68
2. Nigeria	African	400,000	2	0.17	53
3. Singapore	European	15,000	3	5.41	59
	Indian	111,000	1	0.18	49
	Chinese	1,014,000	7	0.14	58
	Malay	190,500	1	0.10	53
4. Fiji	European	7,500	2	7.62	60
	Indian	165,000	2	0.34	51
	Fijian	137,000	1	0.21	32

Source: Kyle et al.[59]

Up till the present it has been postulated by research workers that muscular incoordination of the smooth colonic muscle was at fault.[66, 105] Others also point to other factors than diet that affect bowel movements and lead to constipation.[57] Lack of exercise, poor postural tone, overuse of purgatives, and emotional tension all contribute no doubt to the condition but the overriding cause would seem certain to be a low residue diet on the evidence presented by Painter and Burkitt.

Diverticulosis and diverticulitis are not uncommon conditions in old age (Fig. 10.3). A recent study in England found diverticulae present in one in three persons over the age of 60.[67] Higher incidences than this have been reported.[55]

To clinch his argument that low residue diets cause the

disease and high residue diets prevent it, Painter[79] has successfully treated diverticulitis by a diet high in bran. Of 70 patients with diverticular disease 62 were markedly improved by prescribing a high residue diet. Patients were advised to eat All Bran, Weetabix, Porridge, wholemeal bread, fruit, vegetables, and told to reduce their intake of refined sugar. They were advised to take 2 teaspoonfuls three times a day of unprocessed bran. No patient relapsed while on treatment. Painter and Burkitt conclude that

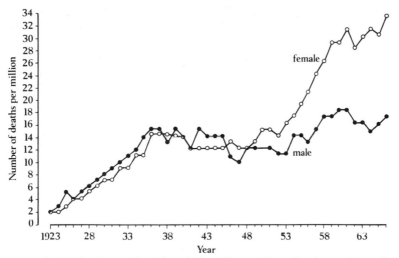

10.3 Crude death rate for diverticular disease (from Registrar General's Statistical Review of England and Wales 1923-66)

diverticular disease is a deficiency disease and like scurvy should be avoided!

Appendicitis

The story is the same with appendicitis. Races civilised have a high incidence of this disease, those uncivilised a low incidence. Some of this difference can be attributed to less efficient medical attention. The large part however derives almost certainly from environmental factors. As also with other diseases considered in this book, a large rise in the frequency of appendicitis occurred at the turn of the century, and this can be correlated with changing food habits.

193

In Asia, Africa and Polynesia and amongst American and West Indian negroes acute appendicitis used to be a rare disease. It is still uncommon where living habits are tribal or primitive and food unsophisticated. In America, though, the Negro is now equalling the white man in frequency of occurrence and in Africa the disease, in the cities, is on the increase. Omo-Dare and Thomas[74] report from Lagos on acute appendicitis and in 1966 record 228 patients admitted for acute appendicitis over a 2-year period. These patients were nearly all Africans living in Lagos, a large proportion of whom came from professional and student classes. Their living habits were westernised. In the villages and country the disease is still comparatively rare.

Striking differences in frequency of appendicitis have been recorded between colonial settlers and natives within certain geographical areas. In pre-war Tunisia, French West Africa, Congo and the Dutch possessions, European and colonial settlers had a greater frequency of the disease as compared to natives.[73, 100] Table 10.2 gives an indication of the difference that existed between British troops resident in India and local Indians, during the last war.

TABLE 10.2

Frequency of Acute Appendicitis in India amongst
native Indian population and resident British
population

Year	Frequency per 1000 population British	Indian
1937	7	1.4
1942	9.2	1.2
1946	5.2	1.6

In 1914 Wilkie[104] had recorded a difference between urbanised cultures and peasant cultures as to frequency of appendicitis. Incidence of appendicitis was 1 per 22,000 amongst Roumanian peasants and 1 per 221 in city dwellers in the same country. Many other examples are listed by Rendle Short[82] and Boyce[10] in their respective books on the subject.

Rendle Short in his *The Causation of Appendicitis*[82] seeks to elucidate the common factor in the civilising process that is causing the rise in appendicitis disease. Though small in volume the book

194

is simply and clearly written and does not attempt to force facts to fit preconceived theories. However Short finally draws the conclusion that the main aetiological factor concerned with the disease is the lack of fibre in modern food. Our contemporary diet is refined and soft and as in diverticulitis presents a viscous non-bulky stool to the intestine. The faeces are propelled sluggishly and with difficulty and predispose to faecolith lodgement within the appendix leading to obstruction and inflammation within that organ.

The vast increase in incidence of appendicitis occurred at the turn of the century and two general practitioners from Ayr in Scotland note the change at the time.[68] Rendle Short gives figures for hospital admissions in the town of Bristol at this period, while Elliot Smith from Oxford shows the very rapid rise in frequency of this disease that occurred in the first 20 years of this century. Elliot Smith is quoted by Cleave and Campbell.[26] His figures show that between 1900 and 1915 recorded cases of appendicitis quadrupled in a British hospital. The pace then slackened off a little and between 1920 and 1940 incidence rose less steeply, fell during the Second World War, rose again in the post-war period and has stabilised since that time.

Rendle Short analyses the changes in diet that occurred at the turn of the century and finds that the most significant changes included:

(1) a large increase in imported foodstuffs: corn, meat, butter, tea, coffee, cocoa, sugar, rice, fruit.
(2) a decrease in consumption of home produced cellulose rich foods: root vegetables (swedes, carrots etc.), leaf vegetables, oatmeal porridge, rye, barley, wholewheat products.
(3) an increase in consumption of processed foods: chocolate, sugar confectioneries, preserved meats, canned vegetables, refined flour products, such as 70% refined white bread and pastries.

The unifying factor that was common to these three changes was a *progressive loss of fibre from food*. A change in consistency in contents of the large bowel was thus argued as predisposing to appendicitis. As the argument put forward is so markedly similar to that propounded in the case of diverticulitis it would be interesting to look at hospital records more closely at that particular time to observe any correlation between the two diseases.

195

To support his theory of causation Rendle Short observes:

(1) That apes in captivity suffer appendicitis and lack a coarse vegetable fibrous diet.

(2) that appendicitis is an urban disease.

(3) that rabbits· when cellulose is eliminated from the diet, incur an inflammation of the caecum that can be remedied by adding horn shavings to the diet.

(4) that the remission of the disease in both World Wars (particularly the second) was accompanied by a roughening and simplification of the diet.

Burkitt[19] postulates that raised intraluminal pressure in the colon following removal of fibre from the diet, is reflected in raised pressures within the appendix particularly when blocked by faecoliths which are peculiar to constipated bowels. Excess sugar alters the bacterial flora which predisposes to E. coli infection and inflammation of the appendix.

One argument against the dietary origins of appendicitis rests upon the fact that constipation is not a regular accompaniment to the disease. Regular bowel movements are often recorded as being present in those afflicted with appendicitis, before onset of the acute phase. The difficulty rests with the defining of constipation. Cleave and Campbell[22] argue that all are constipated who do not have two bowel actions a day! The African apparently has two soft motions each day, the Englishman one sluggish one. Barium meal and follow through studies have been carried out to show this difference. Thus it is argued that a regular bowel movement each day can still be constipation if the stool is hard and its *time of passage through the intestine extra long.*

Other theories concerning origins of appendicitis involve consideration of bacterial infection as a primary factor and also lymphoid hyperplasia. Bacterial infection is probably secondary to faecolith impaction, though it is difficult to prove the exact sequence of events. Lymphoid hyperplasia is a separate and definite aetiology in appendicitis and one that is often found in the case of. children. It is generally associated with lymphatic enlargement elsewhere in the body.

Intestinal stasis can be caused by more than one factor and in summary it is probably true to say that diet as well as other civilising habits including sedentary occupation and lack of exercise play a part in the causation of the disease.[1] The lack of fibre in the food may be shown in time to be of primary importance in aetiology.

Varicose veins and haemorrhoids

Cleave and Campbell[26] claim that varicose veins result from a constipated bowel. They argue that the overloaded colon prolapses
over the left common iliac vein and obstructs venous return. As a
consequence the valvular system of the veins of the lower leg
are stressed and varicosities appear. The caecum likewise by this
theory obstructs the right common iliac vein. The greater frequency
of left leg varicosities as compared to right is explained by the
fact that the colon is distended in constipation and more liable to
prolapse over the iliac vein while the sitting position is being
maintained. Dodd[34] agrees with Cleave and Campbell that diet is
a dominant factor in aetiology.

Others are not so sure and claim other factors as important.
These possible aetiological factors include:

(1) genetic predisposition
(2) obesity
(3) occupation at work that involves standing
(4) pregnancy
(5) multiple arterio-venous fistulae
(6) the wearing of tight garments
(7) lack of exercise
(8) prolonged sitting.

As with other diseases so far mentioned some factor or factors
within our society today are operating to cause this condition.
Many workers[8, 26, 32] have pointed out how rare the disease is in
Africa and yet the Negro in the United States suffers at a level
equal to that of the white man.[62, 94] Barker[8] reports a frequency in
Zululand of five cases seen from amongst 14,000 admissions.
Prevalence of the disease in Britain stands at about 4% in the adult
population, 17% in the elderly female population.[34] Mekky et al.[69]
in a recent survey found 32% of female factory workers in Britain
had varicose veins as compared to only 6% in Egypt.

Hereditary factors play a significant part in the disease and
Dodd[34] claims that 75% of cases have a family history.

In the recent careful survey of this disease carried out by
Mekky et al.,[69] 504 cotton workers in England were compared
to 460 cotton workers in Egypt for prevalence of the disease and
presence of operative environmental factors. The British workers

had a prevalence of 32%, the Egyptians 6%. The British workers were found to stand longer, and also to wear tighter undergarments. These two factors impressively correlated with presence of the condition. Frequency of constipation was the same for both groups and though diet analysis was not detailed the type of food eaten was thought not to play a large part in the disease process. The European women who worked standing had a much higher prevalence of varicose veins than those who sat or walked. Lake et al.[60] in 1942 showed that in a departmental store in New York, 74% of women who stood had varicose veins as against 57% of those who sat. Lack of exercise leads to poor muscular tone in the body of western man, and standing for any length of time is tolerated badly. Poor posture contributes to the problem. Mekky et al.[69] also found that prevalence rose with increasing body weight and obesity predisposed to varicose veins.

Alexander[2] has recently put forward a theory that chair sitting causes varicose veins. He agrees that a factor in the western world must contribute to the increase in varicose veins, and states that the substitution of chair-sitting for ground-sitting is the factor. He has carried out tests and noted that change from chair-sitting to ground-sitting increases transmural pressure in the saphenous veins, the pressure in the vein being increased 2.54 times in the sitting positions. If the colon is constipated, the chair-sitting position allows the colon to press upon the iliac vein to a greater extent and cause rise in leg vein pressure. The two factors could be contributory.

Burkitt[20] shows that varicose veins, deep vein thrombosis, and haemorrhoids, have a common epidemiology and suggests that low fibre diets are the common identifying factor leading to constipation, sluggish colonic contents and raised intracolonic pressures. Whatever the exact mechanism diet almost certainly plays some part in the causation of varicose veins.

Haemorrhoids

In the case of haemorrhoids, it can be said with certainty that constipation is the overriding causative factor. Pressure within the rectum of a constipated faecal mass, at defaecation particularly, gives rise to constriction of the superior haemorrhoidal vein and varicosities result. Graham Stewart[46] closely relates occurrence of haemorrhoids to straining at the stool. Lack of fibre in modern food is the reason for constipation and lack of exercise contributes. Four years ago one survey revealed that 16 to 29% of persons took laxatives to aid defaecation. Native Africans have been shown to pass stools twice a day, the consistency of the stool being soft.[33]

Exercise contributes also to venous return, and is especially important in aiding return of blood to the heart from lower extremities. Venous return from the lower abdomen is almost certainly assisted by such means. Lack of exercise and jobs that entail the maintenance of one posture, sitting or standing for any length of time predispose to constipation. The two factors therefore, consistency of diet and amount of exercise taken would seem to interrelate in the causation of this condition.

Cancer of the colon

Dennis Burkitt[19] in a recent paper on cancer relates this disease and its rising incidence in Western civilised countries to large bowel stasis and the consumption of a low fibre highly processed diet. Radio-opaque markers when swallowed show on X-ray the rate that bowel contents move through the colon and the points of hold-up — the caecum, the right upper flexure and the sigmoid colon — *which are the cancer sites.* It would seem common sense to link bowel stasis, at these points, with irritation of the colonic wall and development of cancer. Burkitt postulates that a carcinogen formed from degradation of bile salts or other bowel constituents is held in contact with the mucosa for a prolonged period in a constipated colon and produces cancer. It has already been shown in this chapter that 'western' stools are less bulky and move much more slowly through the colon (Figs. 10.1 and 10.2).

Hill et al.[52] argue that bile salts are degraded by bacterial flora to produce carcinogens in the colon but say that the extra fat in the 'western' diet is the cause of this particular type of bacterial flora. Burkitt shows that slowed down colonic transit could also lead to greater degradation of bile salts. Aries et al.[6] compare Ugandan stool cultures to Londoners' stools and find distinct differences in flora. The Ugandans in Africa on a vegetarian diet high in bulky fibrous carbohydrates had higher counts of streptococcus and lactobacillus, the Londoners more bacteroids and bifido bacteria. Colonic flora in this manner have a direct bearing upon health.

Gall stones

Another condition where the excessive degradation of bile salts by colonic flora may produce disease is with gall stones. Heaton and Read[51] have shown that malabsorption of bile salts or excessive exposure of bile salts to degradation by intestinal bacteria can lead to upsets in bile resynthesis and the formation of stones.

There are many other factors that could contribute to gall stone disease and it is not the place here to recount these in detail. An alteration in the cholesterol/bile salt ratio in the gall bladder predetermines formation of gall stones and dietary factors can affect this. Possible aetiological factors in gall stone disease are as follows:

High fat diet[39, 103]
High sucrose diet[39, 106]
High meat diet[63, 103]
Low vitamin C intake[41]
Colonic stasis (excess bile degradation)[51]
Obesity[50]
Lack of exercise[84, 107]
Infection and bile stasis[50]

Bacterial flora and E. coli infections

In their book, Cleave and Campbell[26] put forward the theory that diets high in refined carbohydrates predispose to an intestinal colonic floral pattern rich in E. coli organisms. This predominance affects the health of man and causes chronic disease such as pyelonephritis, urinary infection and cholecystitis. The authors again draw upon African data and show the lower incidence of these diseases in rural Africans as opposed to the urbanised. They again point to the fact that the American negro suffers from these diseases at a level more equivalent to the white American.

The link, as yet, is a tenuous one between colonic flora and pyelonephritis and cholecystitis. It is a neat concept to imagine that the type of bacterial population multiplying within the colon determines the type of infective agent found elsewhere within the body but a relatively new concept unbacked by much evidence. Cleave's theory is that the diet rich in refined flour and sugar promotes a flourishing colony of Escherichia Coli in the colon, a gram negative organism which is an unhealthy state, and this unhealthy state promotes infection elsewhere in the body e.g. in the kidney and gall bladder.

It has never been considered seriously that colonic flora might transmit infection to kidney and ureter other than by external contamination but recent work by Schwarz and Seneca does point to a relationship between colonic flora and urinary infection.

Schwarz[86] carried out his experiments at Johns Hopkins Hospital, U.S.A. The right ureter of a dog was ligated to produce hydronephrosis. E. coli obtained from a patient with recurrent urinary infection was then isolated, grown in culture and labelled with radio-active thymidine. The E. coli was also serologically typed. A small area of colonic mucosa in the dog was crushed with forceps and injected with cultured E. coli. The dog was killed and necropsied a day later and the kidneys examined. E. coli of precisely the same variety was identified in the kidneys. Schwarz had shown that E. coli and presumably other bacteria can travel *from colon to kidney* with apparent ease.

Schwarz confirmed his results by typing the E. coli grown from the stools of patients with chronic urinary infection and finding that the variety typed was identical to that in the urine. He then put the theory to practice by putting patients with chronic urinary infections on non-absorbable sulfonamides which destroyed the colonic flora of E. coli and maintained thereby a sterile urine. The need for giving urinary antibiotics in such patients was thus obviated. Treatment of the gut was in effect treatment of the urine.

Seneca et al.[88] give similar clues to the origins of urinary infections and urinary stones by their work on the mucoproteins of stone matrix. Gram negative bacteria such as E. coli in the intestine are known to carry endotoxins in the bacterial cell wall that are both toxic and antigenic in their behaviour. Antibodies are formed against these. When kidney stones form, they form on a focus of inflammation. The mucoprotein of this inflammatory stone material was found to have the same antigen-antibody reaction as the E. coli bacteria in the colon. Seneca et al. were sure that one was closely linked causally with the other and migration had taken place from colon to kidney. They go on to show how E. coli has increasingly dominated urinary infections over the past ten years. However E. coli is not dominant in the gut flora.

The normal flora of the adult human colon is composed of

Bacteroides, Lactobacilli, Diptheroids, Enterococci (e.g. Strep. faecalis), Enterobacilli (e.g. E. coli) and yeast organisms (e.g. Candida albicans). Particular species that appear from time to time include also Proteus, Pseudomonas, Klebsiella, Clostridium perfringens, Shigella and Staphylococcus. Variation of flora is found between individuals and groups of individuals. Although in mice lactobacilli can predominate, in man Bacteroides is the predominant species and can account for up to 90% of bacteria present.[110] E. coli is practically never predominant.

Foods affect intestinal flora but only vague indications exist to date as to the details of these changes. Meat consumption is thought to increase the proportion of coliform organisms and enterococci present,[44] and type of protein is known to affect faecal nitrogen balance probably through bacterial action.[30] The flora also contribute to synthesis of certain B vitamins[54] and a vegetarian diet has been shown to increase this vitamin synthesis.[40, 108, 109] Fats in the diet can increase proportion of Bacteroides present and depress enterococci and lactobacilli[43] though some researches show no effect from the feeding of fat.[38] Cereals[93] increase number of lactobacilli as does the consumption of milk. Yoghurt would seem to affect the amount and type of lactobacilli in the gut also but a fair amount of yoghurt has to be eaten to achieve this and the manner in which the yoghurt is cultivated and fermented affects the results.[48, 85] One type of yoghurt may produce no effect at all. If the yoghurt is rich in lactobacillus bulgaricus it may establish less of an effect as this particular bacillus cannot colonise the human colon. Lactobacillus acidophilus on the other hand can multiply in the human colon and can be ingested as capsules of dry cultures or alternatively introduced into yoghurt.

It has been suggested by *The Lancet*[61] that ingesting cultures of lactobacillus might be a quicker and safer way of dealing with gastroenteritis than customary antibiotic therapy. On the evidence here presented it might also prevent urinary infections.

Dubos and Schaedler[36] have shown in mice how the health, growth and resistance of the species can be affected by the type of colonic flora supported by the animals but no such effect has yet been proved to take place in man. Naturopaths maintain it is so and health food enthusiasts point to the longevity of the Bulgarians as evidence that yoghurt cultures prolong life! However more data is required before one can state a case. Yoghurt has its uses meanwhile in preventing and curing infantile[9] and adult gastro-enteritis[61] and should be used more often for this purpose.

Dental caries and periodontal disease

It would seem unnecessary to prove the point. It has been proved and acknowledged so many times — that the consumption of sticky sweet carbohydrate food promotes dental caries, and encourages poor gum health (periodontal disease). It hardly bears repeating but is testimony enough that our diet should be modified in some way. Even if fluoridation were introduced we should still have the problem of periodontal disease with us and this is as serious a problem as dental caries.

In a recent survey[15] involving Salisbury in Wiltshire and Darlington in the North, 720 subjects were examined for oral health. 82% in Salisbury and 85% in Darlington showed evidence of periodontal disease. 70% showed gingival recession and by the age of 55 none had healthy soft tissues. Two out of three adult persons had partial or complete dentures and two out of five in Salisbury (two out of four in Darlington) had lost all their teeth. Most people examined were unaware of the degree of gum disease present.[16]

Periodontal disease is alarmingly prevalent in this country. Sheiham[89] found 99.7% of school children in a survey in Surrey showed evidence of periodontal disease. Oral cleanliness was poor, and 26% of the 16 year old school children had periodontal pockets (deepened crevices between tooth and gum, associated with loss of alveolar bone). Gingivitis is at the present time the most frequent presentation of periodontal disease and is characterised by redness and swelling of the gums. Gingival recession follows chronic gingivitis or periodontitis and is characterised by recession of the gum from the neck of the tooth with consequent exposure of root surface. The condition leads to eventual loss of teeth.

The principal causes of periodontal disease include: accumulation of food debris around the tooth, calculus, malocclusion, a soft sticky diet, poor dentistry and the presence of dental caries. There is evidence that most of these causes stem from one factor: the type of food we now eat.[14] Raw unprocessed foods such as apples and salads act on the gum tissues by stimulating circulation and encouraging growth of alveolar bone. They have a detergent effect in that they clean away food and are thus an advantage in

203

several respects. Eating apple after meals has been shown to improve oral and dental health.[91]

Malocclusion is also an increasingly modern phenomenon. In this condition the palate is not wide enough to hold the teeth and space them out at regular intervals. Crowding occurs and malformation of tooth development can follow if remedies are not applied. The growth of face, skull and jaw bones are dependent upon hereditary factors and the type of food eaten. Chewing hard and fibrous food promotes growth of bone. In an experiment with rats where soft and hard diets were fed, the soft diet produced a 9 to 13% weaker musculature and 12% less cranium and mandibular bone mass.[70] There was also a decrease of 1 to 2% in the overall size of the brain case. The size of the mandibular angular process (the angle of the jaw bone) was decreased 4% on a soft diet. Barber et al. report similar findings.[7]

Many children today suffer malocclusion in that they have too many teeth for their bone structure. They are unable to shut their mouths properly for discrepancies between size of teeth and size of jaws. D. H. Goose[45] in comparing skulls of the sixth and seventh century with skulls of today has found that a large reduction in palate width has taken place over the years amongst Britons. Change in consistency of diet is thought to be the cause. Whereas tooth size is inherited strongly, palate width is not. Palate width to an extent is acquired by mastication. A child eating a soft diet can therefore not acquire sufficient palate width to carry the teeth. The malocclusion that results accentuates the severity of the periodontal disease. No doubt Weston Price would be happy at this verification of his thesis.

Our modern diets tend to be soft and sticky and designed as one cynic has remarked 'for a nation with ill-fitting dentures'. Much periodontal disease could be prevented by health emphasis upon the need for foods that are fibrous and which require chewing. A diet high in fruit, fresh and raw vegetable and good quality protein would satisfy most demands. By the instituting of such a diet in an experiment with 118 dental students E. Cheraskin[25] produced improvement in health of the gums of the students in four days!

Regarding dental caries the figures tell their own story. In a survey carried out in Salisbury, Wiltshire and Darlington[15] 96% of people with some teeth of their own required dental treatment, as did 90% of those in Darlington. In Salisbury two out of every five adults examined, and in Darlington every other adult, had lost all their teeth. The average adult in Salisbury and Darlington had only 12 and 10 teeth respectively.

In America toothless adult Americans now number more than 20 million and nearly 10 million more have lost either their upper or lower teeth.

Amongst children the tale is as pitiful. *50% of Scottish children of three years of age have tooth decay,* and 95% of children at school leaving age.[83] In Staffordshire from the report of the County School Medical Officer 81% of 5 year olds entering school have tooth decay. Ten years previously this figure was 61%.[4]

A similar situation has been reported by Holloway et al.[53] from dental studies carried out in Tristan da Cunha. Here the introduction into the island of unlimited supplies of refined carbohydrate food resulted in a dental problem for the first time in the island's history. The teeth of the islanders were transformed in quite a short time, from a state of health to a state of widespread disease.

The same rise in incidence of caries found in school children has been chronicled by others[12, 56, 90] and is a sad reflection of the understanding and attention given to dental health by mothers, school teachers, dental authorities and doctors. For the aetiology of dental caries is well known, understood and proved. The Vipeholm experiment in Sweden[47] clinched matters in this regard. The experiment was carried out on prisoners. One group of subjects was given a nutritionally adequate diet low in sugar. Other groups were given the same diet but supplemented with sugar in various forms either as sugar solution or sweets and toffees. The greatest increase in caries occurred in those subjects who consumed sugary confections between meals, which were sticky. Caramels and toffees were more cariogenic than milk chocolate. The most important finding of this study related to the association of between meal consumption of sweets and increase in caries.

Bradford and Crabb[11] also found in children that snacks between meals was the factor that increased caries. Children who abstained from snacks had better oral health. Seventh Day Adventists in Loma Linda, California, abstain from sugar, sticky desserts and highly refined starches. Children belonging to this sect have been observed to have a significantly lower caries rate than neighbouring children in California. Both groups of children reside in non-fluoridated areas.[42]

Almost certainly the eating of sweets, lollipops and snacks has contributed more to the deterioration of children's teeth than any other habit. If nothing else were achieved in the nutritional sphere over the next 50 years but the control of sweet eating and confectionery advertising this would be worth while from the point of view of our children's health. However it is doubtful whether even this can be achieved. What is more sacred, vested financial interests or children's health? In this day and age—the former.

Summary

It is several years now since Surgeon Captain Cleave first published his book with G. D. Campbell, and in the main the arguments put forward in the book have been supported by modern research. Refined carbohydrates and sugar account for many chronic illnesses of our time, particularly diseases of the gastro-intestinal tract as shown in this chapter. Diverticulitis, haemorrhoids, appendicitis, varicose veins and now cancer of the colon have been shown by further evidence to be linked in their aetiology to the eating of such food. Heart diseases, diabetes, and peptic ulcer have a more complicated aetiology and are discussed in separate chapters. Above all, the appalling state of our teeth and our mouths today (periodontal disease) can be straightforwardly attributed to the consumption of a sweet refined diet, as can ordinary obesity and all that follows from this condition. Truly these two groups of foodstuff are to be blamed for much chronic illness today. Is it too much to hope that authoritative measures will be taken in the future to curb the excessive production, advertising and consumption of these foods? Or have we to move further into these areas of illness before enlightenment dawns.

REFERENCES TO CHAPTER 10

1 Aird I., in *Companion to Surgical Studies*, Livingstone, Edinburgh, 1957.
2 Alexander C. J., *The Lancet* 1972, 1:822.
3 Albrink M. J., Lavietes P. H., Man, E. B., *Ann. Intern. Med.* 1963, 58:305.
4 Annual Report of the County School Medical Officer, Staffordshire County Council, 1955.

5 Antar M. A., Ohlson M. A., *J. Nutr.* 1965, 85:329.
6 Aries V., Crowther J. S., Draser B. S., Hill M. J., Williams R., *Gut* 1969, 10:334.
7 Barber C. G., Green L. G., Cox G. J., *J. Dent. Res.* 1963, 42:848.
8 Barker A., *The Lancet* 1964, 2:970.
9 Beck C., Nechelis H., *Amer. J. Gastroent.* 1961, 35:522.
10 Boyce F. F., *Acute Appendicitis and its complications*, Oxford Univ. Press, London 1949.
11 Bradford E. W., Crabb H. S. M., *Brit. Dent. J.* 1961, 111:273.
12 Bransby E. R., Forrest J. R. *Mon-Bull Ministry of Health Lab. Serv.* 1958, 17:28.
13 Braunsteiner H., Herhst M., Sandhopper F., *Germ. Med. Mon.* 1967, 12:426.
14 *Brit. Med. J.* 1965, 2:1197.
15 Bulman J. S., Slack G. L., Richards N. D., Willcocks A. J., *Brit. Dent. J.* 1968, 124:549.
16 ——, ——, ——, ——, *Brit. Dent. J.* 1968, 125:102.
17 Burkitt D. P., *Cancer* 1971, 28:3.
18 ——, *Brit. Med. J.* 1972, 2:556.
19 ——, *The Lancet* 1969, 2:1229.
20 ——, *The Lancet* 1970, 2:1240.
21 Campbell G. D., Cleave T. L., *Brit. Med. J.* 1968, 3:471.
22 ——, ——, *Brit. Med. J.* 1968, 3:741.
23 Carlson A. J., Hoelzel F., *Gastroenterol.* 1949, 12:108.
24 Cheraskin E., Ringsdorf W. M., *J. Med. Ass. State Alabama* 1965, 35:173.
25 ——,*J. Oral Med.* 1966, 21:173.
26 Cleave T. L., Campbell G. D., *Diabetes, Coronary Thrombosis and the Saccharine Disease,* 2nd ed. John Wright, Bristol. 1969.
27 Cohen A. M., Teitelbaum A., Balogh M., Groen J. J., *Amer. J. Clin. Nutr.* 1966, 19:59.
28 Conn J. W., Newburgh L. H., *J. Clin. Invest.* 1936, 15:655.
29 Davidson P., Albrink M. J., *Metabolism* 1965, 14:1059.
30 Deosthale Y. G., Vasantgadkar P. S., Tulpule P. G., *Ind. J. Med. Res.* 1964, 52:111.
31 Devlin J. G., Stephenson N., *Metabolism* 1968, 17:999.
32 Dodd H., *The Lancet* 1964, 2:809.
33 ——, *The Lancet* 1964, 2:910.
34 ——, *Brit. J. Clin. Pract.* 1968, 22:93.
35 Dubos R. J., *'Mirage of Health',* Harper, N.Y. 1959, p.86.
36 Dubos R. J., Schaedler W., *Amer. J. Med. Sci.* 1962, 244:265 and *Fed. Proc.* 1963, 22:1322.
37 Eden M., Phaure T. A., *The Lancet* 1968, 2:264.
38 Frahen H., Greggersen H., Lemke A., Weber E., *Milchwissenschaft* 1966, 21:193.
39 Freston J. W., Bouchier I. A. D., *Gut* 1968, 9:2.
40 Gadziev H. E. K., *Vop Pitan* 1965, 24:19.
41 Ginter E., *The Lancet* 1971, 2:1198.
42 Glass R. L., Hayden J., *J. Dent. Child.* 1966, 33:22.
43 Glatzel H., *Nutritio et Dieta* 1963, 5:192.
44 Goldsmith G. A., *Amer. J. Dig. Dis.* 1965, 10:829.
45 Goose D. H., *World Med.* 1968, 4:no.4, p.63.
46 Graham Stewart C. W., *Dis. Colon & Rectum* 1963, 6:333.

47 Gustaffson B. E., Quensel C. E., Lanke L. S., Lundquist C., Grahnen H., Bonow B. E., *Acta Odont. Scand.* 1953-54, 11:232.
48 Haenel H., Emanuiloff I., Natschef L., Muller W. *Milchwissenschaft* 1963, 18:454.
49 Hales C. N., Greenwood F. C., Mitchell F. L., Strauss W. T., *Diabetologia* 1968, 4:73.
50 Harding Rains A. J., *Gallstones*, Heinemann Medical, London 1964.
51 Heaton K. W., Read A. E., *Brit. Med. J.* 1969, 3:494.
52 Hill M. J., Crowther J. S., Drasar B. S., Hawksworth G., *The Lancet* 1970, 1:95.
53 Holloway P. J., James P. M. C., Slack G. L., *Brit. Dent. J.* 1963, 115:19.
54 Hotzel D., Barnes R. H., *Vitamins & Hormones* 1966, 24:121.
55 Hughes L. E., *Brit. Med. J.* 1968, 1:58.
56 James P. M. C., Parfitt G. J., *Brit. Dent. J.* 1957, 103:214.
57 Jones F. A., Godding E. W., *Brit. Med. J.* 1972, 2:651.
58 Kuo P. T., Bassett D., *Ann. Intern. Med.* 1965, 62:1199.
59 Kyle J., Adesola A. O., Tinckler L. F., De Beaux J. *Scan J. Gastroent.* 1967, 2:77.
60 Lake M., Pratt G. H., Wright I. S., *J. Amer. Med. Ass.* 1942, 119:696
61 *The Lancet* 1970, 2:1169.
62 Lewis J. H., *The Biology of the Negro*, Chicago Univ. Press, Chicago 1942.
63 Lichtmann S. S., *Diseases of the Liver, Gallbladder and Bile Ducts*, 3rd ed. Henry Kimpton, London 1953, p.1297.
64 Luft R., Cerasi E., Madison L. L., Von Euler U.S., Casa L. D., Roovete A., *The Lancet* 1966, 2:254.
65 Macdonald I., Braithwaite D. M., *Clin. Sci.* 1964, 27:23.
66 Manousos O. N., Truelove S. C., Lumsden K., *Brit. Med. J.* 1967, 3:760.
67 ——, ——, ——, *Brit. Med. J.* 1967, 3:762.
68 McKerrow G., Geikie J. S., *Practitioner* 1909, 82:391.
69 Mekky S., Schilling R. S. F., Walford J., *Brit. Med. J.* 1969, 2:591.
70 Moore W. J., *J. Zool.* 1965, 146:123.
71 Mosenthal H. O., Barry E., *Ann. Intern. Med.* 1950, 33:1175.
72 Morgan M. N., Ellis H., *Brit. Med. J.* 1969, 2:53.
73 Muller S., *Acta Chir. Scand.* 1956, suppl. 221:1.
74 Omo-Dare P., Orishejolomi-Thomas H., *W. Afr. Med. J.* 1966, 15:217.
75 Painter N. S., *Amer. J. Dig. Dis.* 1968, 13:468.
76 ——, Truelove S. C., *Gut* 1964, 5:201, 365, 369.
77 ——, Ardran G. M., Tuckey M., *Gut* 1965, 6:57.
78 ——, Burkitt D. P., *Brit. Med. J.* 1971, 2:450.
79 ——, Almeida A. Z., Colebourne K. W., *Brit. Med. J.* 1972, 2:137.
80 Peters N., Hales C. N., *The Lancet* 1965, 1:1144.
81 Refkind B. M., Gale M., Lawson D., *Cardiovasc Res.* 1968, 2:143.
82 Rendle Short A., *The Causation of Appendicitis* John Wright, Bristol 1946.
83 Report of Health and Welfare Services in Scotland, Scottish Home & Health Dept. 1962.
84 Rolleston H., McNee J. W., *Disease of the Liver, Gallbladder and Bile Ducts*, MacMillan, London 1929.
85 Schmidt B., *Med. Ernahrung* 1965, 6:111.
86 Schwarz H., *Med. News* May 6, 1969, p.56.

[87] Seltzer H. S., Fajans S. S., Conn J. W., *Diabetes* 1956, 5:437.
[88] Seneca H., Lattimer J. K., Peer P., *J. Urol.* 1964, 92:603.
[89] Sheiham A., *Dent. Practit.* 1969, 19:232.
[90] Slack G. L., *Brit. Med. J.* 1955, 1:260.
[91] ——, Martin W. J., *Brit. Dent. J.* 1958, 105:366.
[92] Smelo L. S., *Modern Treatment* 1966, 3:342.
[93] Smith H. W., *J. Path. Bact.* 1965, 89:95.
[94] Stamler J., *J. Nat. Med. Ass.* 1958, 50:161.
[95] Stout R. W., Vallance Owen J. *The Lancet* 1969, 1:1078.
[96] Swan D. C., Davidson P., Albrick M. J., *The Lancet* 1966, 1:60.
[97] Szanto S., *The Lancet* 1967, 2:260.
[98] Uram J. A., Friedman L., Kline O. L., *Amer. J. Phys.* 1958, 192:521.
[99] Vallance Owen J., *Quart J. Med.* 1965, 34:485.
[100] Van Ouwerkerk L. W., *Acta. Chir. Neerl.* 1951, 3:164.
[101] Viel B., Donoso S., Salcedo D., *Arch. Intern. Med.* 1968, 122:97.
[102] Welborn T. A., Breckenridge A., Rubinstein A. H., Dollery C. T., Fraser T. R., *The Lancet* 1966, 1:1336.
[103] Wheeler M., Hills L. L., Laby B., *Gut* 1970, 11:430.
[104] Wilkie D. P. D., *Brit. Med. J.* 1914, 2:959.
[105] Williams I., *Gut* 1968, 9:498.
[106] Wright A., Whipple G. H., *J. Exp. Med.* 1934, 59:411.
[107] Yagi T., *Tohoku J. Exp. Med.* 1961, 72:117.
[108] Yamaguchi T., Yano M., Fujita A., *J. Vitaminol* (Kyoto) 1959, 5:88.
[109] Yano M., Fujita A., J. *Vitaminol* (Kyoto) 1958, 4:81.
[110] Zubrzycki L., Spaulding E. H., *J. Bacteriol.* 1962, 83:968.

Eleven

Obesity

The high prevalence of obesity in the western world is due to the following factors:

(1) Palatability: Food is palatable and sweet. The refining of carbohydrates contributes to this.

(2) Wealth: Too much food is eaten for the amount of energy expended. Less exercise is taken.

(3) Psychology: Depression and anxiety can both induce over-eating.

(4) Upbringing: Babies are fed more cereal foods and sugar than before and at an earlier date. It has been shown that obesity in infancy induces obesity in adult life.

(5) Environment: Advertising stresses the need to eat more and to eat the sugar-containing high calorie foods.

Only in rare cases is obesity 'glandular', though heredity plays its part, as is shown later. Small even trivial differences in digestion and absorption between one individual and another can lead to large differences overall in body weight, and the production of obesity.[2] Metabolic factors can play a part in the predisposition to obesity.[32] However, overall calorie excess produces obesity, and overall calorie restriction cures it.[19]

Obesity shortens life, and increases liability to degenerative diseases of the heart, blood vessels, kidney, gall bladder, and induces such disease as diabetes and arthritis.[17] It has been termed our main affluent disease.

Prevalence
20% - 30% of young men and women are overweight and 50% of those over 40 years of age.[30] Prevalence of obesity within the
210

general population probably rests at about 20% at the present time, using the usual diagnostic parameter of weight for height.[14, 29, 33]

In America insurance statistics show similar percentages for incidence of obesity in the general population.[39] 20% of men were overweight and 10% were severely overweight. In the 30-39 age group 50% of men were overweight. In the 50-59 age group 60% were overweight and half of these were severely overweight.

Obesity carries an increased mortality and a predisposition to degenerative disease.[39] Excess mortality for men 20% overweight is a third greater than normal. It is less marked for women. Excess mortality is greatest in regard to diabetes (130% increase in mortality) nephritis (70% increase) diseases of the digestive system (70% increase) cerebral vascular accidents (50% increase in mortality) and heart disease (40% increase in mortality). Other hazards the obese must face[5, 11, 27, 34] include high blood pressure, complications of pregnancy, osteoarthritis, gout, bronchitis, increased incidence of cancer and premature death! Sinclair has laconically remarked that to be 10 lbs. overweight carries a greater health risk than to smoke 25 cigarettes a day.

Heredity

Food is plentiful and we eat more of it than we should and yet some become more obese than others. The fact was commented upon by Dr. Johnson. Johnson in Boswell's memoirs[4] was 'talking of a man who had grown very fat so as to be incommoded with corpulency'. Johnson remarked:

> 'He eats too much, Sir'.
>
> Boswell: 'I don't know Sir; you will see one man fat who eats moderately, and another lean who eats a great deal'.
>
> Johnson: 'Nay, Sir, whatever maybe the quantity that a man eats it is plain that if he is too fat, he has eaten more than he should have done. One man may have a digestion that consumes food better than common; but it is certain that solidity is increasedly putting something to it!'

However much one admires Johnson's forceful logic, if one comes from a fat family one's chances of becoming fat are much higher than normal. Mayer[28] shows from a survey of 15 year olds in Boston that with parents of normal weight 10% of the children are likely to be overweight. If one parent is obese, 40% of the children are likely to be overweight, while if both parents are obese there is an 80% chance that the children will be so too. Thus Boswell was right in that inherent tendencies play a part in the development of obesity. Johnson was correct too however in stressing that obesity cannot be present in the absence of an abundance of food. Nowhere is this more important perhaps than in childhood.

Infancy and childhood

Overfeeding in infancy is one of the most important factors pre-disposing to adult obesity.[6] Widdowson and McCance[40] found that rats which were overfed with milk during the first 20 days of life (equivalent to a year or more of a baby's life) grew into heavier animals than those which received limited amounts of food in the first 20 days. A correlation has also been reported between weight in infancy and weight at five years old; the more overweight the baby the more overweight the five year old.[41] This correlation has now been shown to carry through to adulthood.[23, 20] Fat babies make fat men. Kemp[18] found that 40% of obese adults were obese in childhood. Another 14% started their obesity in early adult life (associated with such factors as less exercise, beer drinking, early marriage etc.). In 30% of cases obesity followed childbirth, and in 31% it followed inactivity in middle age.

Infants are overweight from overfeeding and from the particular type of feeding that is current nowadays. Sweetened infant foods are the rule rather than the exception. Breast milk contains no added sugar! Breast feeding unfortunately however is unpopular. Normal satiety responses are disturbed following ingestion of oversweetened foods and infants (like experimental rats) can be plied with such foods till they become obese. Mothers tend to overfeed for a number of reasons. In many cases no doubt there is ignorance. In other instances an unnatural preoccupation exists concerning the weight of the baby. The weighing scales become the most important item in the house. Psychologically also it suits many mothers to overfeed. Apley and Keith[3] define in this context an 'umbilical cord syndrome', where the wish on the part of the mother to maintain an abnormally close relationship with the baby stems from a need for comfort and security. Feeding the baby is used as the means of maintaining this relationship and

212

extra food a means of confirming it. Infant obesity is a likely result. However perspective is always necessary in dealing with such problems and many would hold in this instance that a loved and happy infant however obese is preferable to an unloved infant of normal weight! Theoretical though this choice of alternatives may be it is necessary to point out again that infant obesity predisposes to adult obesity which predisposes to disease and it should be avoided.

School children are heavier and taller today than ever before.[13] Weight however is increasing proportionately faster than height. There are more fat children at school than before. Scott[37] in a London County Council survey of heights and weights of school-children, showed that between 1949 and 1959, girls between 11 and 12 increased their average weight by 3.05 kg (6.6 lb) or 8.5% and their height by 3 cm or 2.1%. Weight thus increased far more than height. This was so for all age groups of both sexes and was found excessively to be the case in the 90th percentile of weight distribution. This refers to the 10% of children who were the heaviest of each group. Obesity had increased by a larger amount in this group. The annual reports of the Chief Medical Officer of the Ministry of Education for the years 1956-57, 1960-61 and 1964-65[35] comment upon the increasing prevalence of obesity in school children.

P. M. Mortimer[31] in a recent survey of obesity in a secondary girls' school in Croydon, Surrey, compared her findings with Scott's findings in 1959 and found that for mean weight there had been an increase in the girls of 5.9% - 15.6% but for height a 1.98% - 3.02% increase. A total of 8% of the girls were now found definitely to be obese and successful dieting was carried out for this group. Whether they eat more at Croydon than at Leicester or whether classification of obesity was less strict in Leicester, recent findings in that city point to only 3% of children as being obese.

In America the problem is a bigger one. Numerous surveys have now been carried out on teenagers and whereas ten years ago estimates of obesity averaged about 10%[21] in teenage surveys, Dwyer et al.[10] now find that 15.2% of young teenagers are obese and Canning et al.[8] 23.3% in one survey. Amongst boys alone estimates show that 11% to 14% of boys are so afflicted.[15] These obese children also eat badly, consuming deficient diets.[16, 38]

213

Foods

Any food taken in excess will produce obesity. Calories put on weight if not burnt up and used by the body. Carbohydrates and sugar particularly, provide rapidly absorbed calories and can lead therefore to a speedy accumulation of body fat if not utilised in some other manner by the body. Fatstock farmers are aware of this fact in animal husbandry. Sucrose and carbohydrates therefore are often named as the cause of all obesity. They are not the exclusive cause. Fats can produce obesity and proteins can. All that is required to produce obesity is a body intake and absorption of food greater than body requirement where means are not available for using up the calories in external work or respiration. Sucrose[1] and carbohydrates[24, 25, 26] indeed put on fat. Fats[12, 21, 22] have also been shown to do so and Lemonnier[22] shows a certain potentiation between these two foodstuffs in increasing body weight. Foods which are eaten in abundance in the western world and which contribute to obesity, generally contain all three elements — fat, carbohydrate and protein. Such foods would include snack foods, pastry foods, cakes, biscuits etc. Sugar of course is also taken in its purified and concentrated form and contributes substantially to obesity.

The balance of foods that go to make up a total diet are however important and Larsson[21] has shown in his experiments on fat intake and obesity that this is so. Larsson was concerned to show the effect of fat upon obesity and fed mice three different diets. Diet A was composed of nutrients as found in a normal Swedish diet. Diet B was the diet recommended by the country's National Institute of Public Health for public consumption. Diet C was a diet very high in fat, and very low in carbohydrate. Table 11.1 sets out the diets. It is noted that sucrose was excluded from all three diets.

All three diets were iso-caloric but diets A, the Swedish diet, and C, the high fat diet led to obesity while B did not. Diet A gave 28% fat content of carcass. Diet C gave 36% fat content of carcass and Diet B gave 21%. Larsson recommends on this and other experiments that one should reduce intake of fat (and sucrose) and increase intake of skim milk, bread, potatoes, vegetables. The National Swedish Institute of Public Health in promoting Diet B, the diet that Larsson recommends, had done so for the reason that authorities were concerned over falling Swedish consumption of fruit, vegetables, potatoes and bread and the way this consumption was being replaced by sucrose, fat and processed foods. The same story, told once again!

TABLE 11.1

Composition of the three diets used by Larsson in experiments on obesity

Diet A: a normal Swedish diet
Diet B: recommended by Nat. Inst. Public Health, Sweden
Diet C: a high fat diet

| | *DIETS* | | |
	A.	B.	C.
Foods	g	g	g
Vegetables **	2.8	4.6	4.0
Fruits, berries	12.5	15.4	15.4
Potatoes	17.1	19.1	2.0
Bread, cereals	14.6	22.3	0
Milk, cheese	29.5	29.6	29.6
Meat, fish, egg	12.8	10.5	35.5
Fat (butter etc.)	3.7	2.2	11.5
Calories per g *	1.8	1.6	2.1

* cellulose was added to give 1.6 cal/g, and all diets made iso-caloric.
** Green vegetables 65%, dried peas beans 35%.

Two other factors in the causation of obesity are worth attention. The first is lack of exercise. Lack of activity besets many of us in our modern living and it has been shown by Mayer[28] that the obese take less exercise than others and are inactive people. It has also been shown that obese children expend less energy than non obese[7] and in one survey of obese children during the day and throughout the night, the immobility of the obese child was quite striking.[36] However it is difficult for the overweight to lose their weight by exercise for exercise is difficult if one is obese!

Summary
There is an urgent need for sound nutritional education of mother and child at the present time. Obesity is now presenting as a real threat to health. Sugar should not be fed to babies and the early feeding of cereals to babies withheld. Advertising of sweets should also be drastically curbed. If television remains the measure

The food and health of western man

of our health education the outlook is grim. At the present time one can say a child is manipulated by these persuasive measures to be ill. This is hardly right in this enlightened age.

REFERENCES TO CHAPTER 11

1 Allen R. J. L., Leahy J. S., *Brit. J. Nutr.* 1966, 20:339.
2 Anderson J., *Brit. Med. J.* 1972, 1:560.
3 Apley J., Keith R. M., *The Child and his Symptoms, a Psychosomatic Approach,* Blackwell, Oxford 1962.
4 Boswell J., *Life of Johnson,* Charles Dilly, London 1791.
5 *Brit. Med. J.* 1963, 2:764.
6 Brooke C. G. D., Lloyd J. R., Wolf O. H., *Brit. Med. J.* 1972, 1:25.
7 Bullen, B. A., Reed R. B., Mayer J., *Amer. J. Clin. Nutr.* 1964, 14:211.
8 Canning H., Mayer J., *Postgrad Med.* 1965, 38:A.101.
9 Dublin L. I., Marks H. H., *Proc. Ass. Life Insur. Med. Directors of America* 1951, 4.
10 Dwyer J. T., Feldman J. J., Mayer J., *Amer. J. Clin. Nutr.* 1967, 20:1045.
11 Emerson R. G., *Brit. Med. J.* 1962, 2:516.
12 Fabrỳ P., Braun T., Petrasck R., *Physiol. Bohemoslov* 1964 13:333.
——Hejda S., Cerny K., *Amer. J. Clin. Nutr.* 1966, 18:358.
13 Garn S. M., Haskell J. A., *Amer. J. Dis. Child.* 1960, 99:746.
14 Hopkins P., *The Practitioner* 1965 194:150.
15 Huenemann R. L., *Amer. J. Clin. Nutr.* 1966, 18:325.
16 ——Hampton M. C., Shapiro L. R., *Fed. Proc.* 1966, 25:4.
17 ——*Publ. Health Rept.* 1968, 83:49.
18 Johnson M., Burke B., Mayer J., *Amer. J. Clin. Nutr.* 1956, 4:231.
19 Kemp R., *The Practitioner* 1966, 196:404.
20 Kinsell L. W., Gunning B., Michaels G. D., Richardson J., *Metabolism* 1964, 13:195.
21 Larsson S., *Acta Phys. Scand.* 1967, suppl. 294, 'Factors for the etiology of obesity in mice'.
22 Lemonnier D., *Cahiers Nutr. Dietétique* 1967, 2:29 (*Nutr. Abst. Rev.* 1968. 2872).
23 Lloyd J. K., Wolff O. H., Whelan W. S., *Brit Med. J.* 1961, 2:145.
24 Litwack G., Hankes L. V., Elvehjem C. A., *Proc. Soc. Exp. Biol. Med.* 1952, 81:441.
25 MacDonald I., *J. Physiol. Lond.* 1962, 162:334.
26 ——*World Rev. Nutr. Dietet.* 1967, 8:143.
27 Marks H. H., *Bull. N.Y. Acad. Med.* 1960, 36:296.
28 Mayer J., *Med. Clin. N. Amer.* 1965, 49:421.
29 McMullan J. J., *The Practitioner* 1959, 182:222.
30 Montegriffo V. M. F., *Ann. Hum. Gen.* 1968, 31:389.
31 Mortimer P. M., *Proc. Nutr. Soc. Lond.* 1968, 27:29.
32 Pawan G. L. S., *Med. News Tribune,* Aug. 13, 1971.
33 Pincherle C., Wright H. B., *J. Coll. Gen. Pract.* 1967, 13:280.
34 Planchu M., *J. de Med. de Lyon* 1865, 46:1147. (World wide abstr. 1966 9:40).
35 Report of the Chief Med. Offr. Ministry of Educ. *Health of the School Child,* 1956-57, 1960-61, 1964-65. H.M.S.O. 1958, 1962, 1966.
36 Rose G. A., Williams R. T., *Brit. J. Nutr.* 1961, 15:1.

216

[37] Scott J. A., *Report on Heights and Weights of School Pupils in County of London,* 1954 publ. L.C.C. 1955.

[38] Shapiro L. R., Hampton M. C., Huenemann R. L., *J. Sch. Health* 1967 37:166.

[39] Society of Actuaries *Build and Blood Pressure Study* publ. Soc. Actuaries, Chicago 1960.

[40] Widdowson E. M., McCance R. A., *Proc. Roy. Soc. Biol.* 1960, 152: 188.

[41] Wolff O. H., *Triangle* 1966, 7:234.

Twelve

Diabetes

Maturity onset diabetes is another degenerative disease of the human body found increasingly within western civilisation, and associated with western ways of living and eating.

The one factor that is overrulingly associated with diabetes is that just discussed—obesity.[34] The obese individual is liable to diabetes. Control his obesity and his diabetes is similarly controlled. These are facts now well established, so well established that a campaign could well be mounted in this country similar to the smoking and lung cancer campaign to curb obesity and so reduce the incidence of diabetes, if it was the real wish of the profession or the public, (which is in doubt).

For the evidence West and Kalbfleisch[61] have examined age matched groups and representative population samples from Chinese in Malaya, Pakistanis in East Pakistan, Negroes in Central America, Caucasian whites in Central South and North America, and have noted large differences in overall prevalence. But when races and populations were matched for obesity the differences were small. It is recognised that there are racial and genetic factors[5, 42] affecting the incidence of this disease but the overruling *environmental* factor is obesity in all these studies. The genetic factor contributing to diabetes, (the juvenile onset type particularly) accounts for the mention of this disease as far back as 1500 B.C. In fact Hindu, Chinese and Japanese writers over a thousand years have given accounts of diabetes.

The factors therefore responsible for this disease in the western world are factors which contribute to obesity; increased palatability of food, increased intake of a rich, refined diet, high in calories, leading to general overnutrition which against a background of

218

inactivity and less exercise gives rise to obesity.

Incidence and geographical distribution

A recent survey of the prevalence of diabetes in this country in the town of Bedford[9] showed that 12 - 14% of the adult population possessed an abnormal glucose tolerance test, indicative of overt or incipient diabetes. It has been shown that a significant number of these latent diabetics at a further stage develop diabetes.[5] This was a sophisticated and careful survey and revealed a quantity of diabetes within the population not before suspected. A survey in America using glucose tolerance analysis similarly uncovered prevalence estimates of 10%. This is confirmed by other findings.[44]

The Office of Health Economics in their survey show a *tenfold* increase in registered diabetics between 1941 and 1962.[45] Some of this rise can be put down to keener diagnosis and better medicine. A lot cannot. It has been forecast that in the next 20 years the prevalence could increase two to threefold, resulting in a 30% prevalence of the disease throughout the country!

Prevalence estimates throughout the world vary very much according to racial susceptibility, obesity, diet (western or native) and type of analysis procedure undertaken (urine analysis, random blood sugars or glucose tolerance studies). Amongst the Indians of Alaska[41] and the Eskimoes[42] the disease is rare. However amongst other native Americans influenced by western dietary factors the prevalence of diabetes is very high indeed. The Seneca,[21] Cherokee[55] and Cocopah Indians[28] have prevalence rates in the adult of 22%, 31% and 34% respectively, whilst the American Pima Indians[3] lead the field with a prevalence rate of 50% in those over 35 years of age! The Pima Indians are in general obese and consume a diet very high in calories, derived from a combination of native and western food.[50] It would seem that certain uncivilised people are more than usually susceptible to western degenerative diseases when they become civilised. One can foresee in the future a huge increase in certain diseases as the luxuries of western living spread round the globe! It has been shown for instance that Indians crossing over to Natal develop it,[14, 63] Zulus coming to the town environment develop it[10] and the Bantu in becoming urbanised becomes prone to it.[48, 52] Others have shown also the correlation between urbanisation and onset of diabetes.[8, 30, 43]

The Polynesians in the South Pacific have proved interesting material for the study of the relationship of environment and disease and Prior et al.[49] have shown that the New Zealand Maoris who are of Polynesian descent have a much higher incidence of the disease than their purer cousins who have remained on the island of Puka-Puka in the South Pacific. The Maoris suffer diabetes at an 8% prevalence level, the Puka Pukans at a 1.3% level. The Maoris have a westernised diet consuming 71 g of sucrose a day. The Puka Pukans live off fish, taro and coconut, 9 g of sugar and have a lower overall calorie consumption. Other diseases of civilisation found in the Maoris include obesity, hypertension, heart disease and perhaps gout.[38, 49] Difference in consumption of sugar was marked between the two races.

Overnutrition and obesity is not only a matter of sugar consumption though this is a potent causal factor. Sugar is incriminated, by Cohen and his workers[15, 19] in Israel. Yemenites migrating to Israel from the Yemen become susceptible to diabetes over a certain period of time. At home their frequency of diabetes is 0.06%. In Israel it rises to 2.6%. The principal difference in diet is a drop in the consumption of bread and an increase in sugar.[16] Sugar intake increased from 6 g to 60 g a day. A small increase in calories was noted and marginal increase in obesity. Animal fat consumption could not account for disease increase in this case.

The Indian in South Africa on the other hand has increased his consumption of both fat and sugar together with calorie intake in general. Booyens and De Waal[6] show that carbohydrates are consumed almost exclusively in the refined form, white bread, polished rice and flour. His fat consumption now provides some 30-40% of calorie intake whereas before it provided some 5-10%. His sugar intake has trebled and more. Prevalence of diabetes in India in the population is estimated by Cleave and Campbell at 1% (only an approximate figure) whereas in Natal it is estimated at 2.3% in village dwellers and 5.2% in better off urbanised Indians.[10, 14] Glucose Tolerance testing has revealed the incredibly high figure of 37% of the Indian population in Natal as suffering from abnormal findings suspicious of latent diabetes![14] This particular race thus seems overly sensitive to the development of the disease. Fat, sugar and calories probably all contribute in this case.

The same trend in change in eating habits is occurring in other parts of Africa.[10, 26, 48, 52]

The pathogenesis of diabetes
Joslin shows in his well-known book *The Treatment of Diabetes* the correlation that exists between obesity and diabetes.[31]

Correlation between obesity and diabetes

Amount Overweight	Increase in Diabetic Mortality above that of men of normal weight
5-15%	$1\frac{1}{2}$
15-24%	$3\frac{1}{2}$
25%	$8\frac{1}{3}$

To him who has the diabetic tendency it is therefore unwise to become overweight. 'Gorging' is also a mistake! Fabry[25] and now many other workers have shown that eating large meals carries with it a risk of metabolic stress. Large heavy meals cause hyperglycemia and require a large insulin output. They also predispose to obesity. Houssay and Martinez[29] in their now classical series of experiments showed that 'gorging' rats were inclined to diabetes. Mosinger et al.[40] showed that such rats had an output of insulin far higher than normal and as a result were depleted of insulin reserves.

Obesity on its own however does not always cause diabetes.[53] Some obese are therefore more prone than others. It has been suggested that overnutrition, the cause of obesity, stimulates the production of insulin from the pancreas to the point of exhaustion. The cells of the pancreas degenerate, the insulin levels drop and diabetes results. Confirmation is given to this 'exhaustion theory' by the fact that an obese diabetic can often control the disease by losing weight and eating less. The stress is thus removed from the pancreas and homeostasis restored in such cases. All obese individuals secrete a greater amount of insulin following food intake than their lean counterparts.[47] They have thus an oversecretion which is perhaps a prelude to exhaustion. The obese that become diabetic probably have a deficiency of pancreatic cell structure in addition which finally leads to the development of diabetes. Recent studies on insulin secretion in some of the mildest of diabetics have shown that the ß cells of the pancreas are poorly regulated and produce but a slow rise of circulating insulin in response to a carbohydrate meal.[4, 13] There is a structural defect therefore which could be linked by some theories to autoimmune mechanisms. Juvenile diabetics have little or no insulin in the circulating blood.[33]

Animal experiments reveal that high fat, high carbohydrate or high protein diets can all predispose to diabetes if the calorie intake is excessive[29] (Table 12.1). Other workers have shown the potent diabetogenic effect of concentrated glucose feeding in cats.[2, 7, 22, 23, 56]

TABLE 12.1
Diabetic Mortality in alloxan treated rats, on different diets[29]

Diet	% Composition			% Mortality
	Wheat & Corn Flour	Casein	Fat	
High starch	69	20		40
High protein	44	45		33
High lard	35	20	34	100
High butter	35	20	34	33
High olive oil	35	20	34	40
High corn oil	35	20	34	13
Low protein, high starch	79	10		90

Source: Houssay B. A., Martinez, C. *Science* 1947, 105: 548.

Uram et al.[57] in more sophisticated experiments differentiated between a cereal diet, a sucrose diet and a lard (animal fat) diet in their effect upon glucose tolerance in the rat (see Fig. 12.1). The cereal diet produced less pathological change in the animals. In their conclusions Uram et al. consider the cereal diet to be healthier for reasons of its slower digestibility and absorption. These workers note that at the turn of the century, Von Noorden[59] an authority on diabetes at that time, had popularised the use of oatmeal diets in the treatment of diabetes, having found this a successful therapy in the disease.

It would seem from the evidence so far presented, *that over-*

nutrition and that derived particularly from the consumption of fats, sugars and refined carbohydrates is the most important nutritional aetiological factor in maturity onset diabetes.

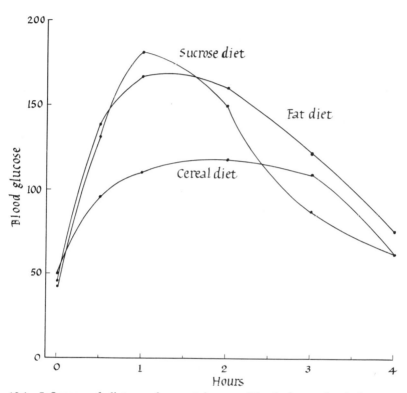

12.1 Influence of diet on glucose tolerance. Blood glucose levels in rats are shown following a glucose loading test, the rats having been fed on three different diets (from Uram J. A., Friedman L., Kline O. L., *Amer. J. Physiol.* 1958, 192:521)

With many foods as they are eaten today, sucrose and butter, or sucrose in combination with some other fat, are frequent constituents. Pastry, cake, biscuit, chocolates, ice cream all contain combinations of these two elements and sucrose and butter are common elements in themselves at most meals. The story has been told in the previous chapter on heart disease and is basically similar here. These two food stuffs, simple carbohydrate and animal

223

fat, can potentiate each other in their effect upon blood triglyceride levels,[11, 36] blood cholesterol,[37] liver fat,[12] and overall body weight.[35] Increase in body weight and alteration in blood sugar homeostasis are the two effects pertinent to the pathogenesis of diabetes. There is evidence from the experiments of Lemonnier[35] and Uram et al.[57] that animal fat and sucrose can act synergistically here too. In view also of the fact that both substances have been incriminated in heart disease and diabetes it is interesting and not surprising that both diseases are often found in the same person.[20] There is three or four times as much coronary artery disease amongst diabetics as controls[27] and 75% of patients after a heart attack show abnormal glucose tolerance tests,[54] an impairment which lasts many months.[18]

TABLE 12.2

Diets used in the experiments by Uram et al.[57] on glucose tolerance testing in rats. gm/100 gm

Cereal diet		Sucrose diet		Fat diet	
Yellow corn meal	73.6	Sucrose	66.0	Sucrose	32.8
Ground barley	3.3	Casein	20.8	Casein	27.0
Linseed meal	5.0	Lard	3.8	Lard	27.9
Wheat	7.3	Cotton seed oil	1.2	Cotton seed oil	1.56
Oat flour	5.0	Cysteine	0.2	Cysteine	0.26
Dried skim milk	4.0	Salts	4.0	Salts	5.19
Blood flour	1.0	Flour & vitamins	4.0	Flour & vitamins	5.19
Salt vitamins	.8				

Source: Uram J. A., Friedman L., Kline O. L., *Amer. J. Physiol.* 1958, 192:521.

To make the final point, there is an interesting case report of a 19-year-old boy[1] who ate excessively and developed diabetes. The boy ate three generous meals a day in addition to a big intake of chocolates, candy, malted milk, soda pop and snacks. His calorie intake was 7000 cals/day, four sevenths of which was derived from carbohydrate! Dieted and given insulin his condition so much improved that after six months he was taken off insulin, on the whole an unwise action as the boy grew careless, reverted to his old eating habits and again developed severe diabetes.

If overeating causes diabetes, undereating should prevent it. Undereating is certainly an effective method of treating diabetes and the diet should be low in refined carbohydrates and high in good protein, fruit and vegetable. Kempner[32] treated his diabetics with rice and fruit diets. A less extreme cereal, fruit and vegetable diet is advocated by Ernest and co-workers.[24] They recommend an intake of 150 g of bread, 200 g of potato, fruit, vegetable and a pint of skimmed milk a day. The diet is low in both sucrose and fat, and leads to stabilised insulin levels, lowered cholesterol levels and improvement in vascular lesions. Van Noorden suggested a similar type of diet many years previously.[58, 60]

REFERENCES TO CHAPTER 12

1 Alpert S., *Ann. Intern. Med.* 1955, 42:927.
2 Barron S. S., State D., *Arch. Path.* 1949, 48:297.
3 Bennett P. H., Burch T. A., Miller M., *The Lancet* 1971, 2:125.
4 Berson S. A., Yalow R. S., *Amer. J. Med.* 1961, 31:874.
5 Birmingham Diabetes Survey Working Party, *Brit. Med. J.* 1970, 3:301.
6 Booyens J., DeWaal V. M., *S. Afr. Med. J.* 1970, 44:1415.
7 Brown E. M., Dohan F. C., Freedman L. R., DeMoor P., Lukens F. D. W., *Endocrinol.* 1952, 50: 644.
8 Brunner D., Altman S., Nelken L., Reider J., *Diabetes* 1964 13:268.
9 Butterfield W. J., *Proc. Roy. Soc. Med.* 1964, 57:195.
10 Campbell G. D., *S. Afr. Med. J.*, 1963, 37:1199.
11 Carroll C., *J. Nutr.* 1963, 79:93.
12 ——Bright E., *J. Nutr.* 1965, 87:202.
13 Cerasi E., Luft R., *Acta Endocrinol.* 1967. 55:278.
14 Cleave T. L., Campbell G. D., *Diabetes, Coronary Thrombosis and the Saccharine Diseases,* J. Wright, Bristol, 2nd ed. 1969.
15 Cohen A. M., *Metabolism* 1961, 10:50.
16 ——Bavly S., Poznanski R., *The Lancet* 1961, 2:1399.
17 ——Teitelbaum A., *Amer. J. Physiol.* 1964, 206:105.
18 ——Shafrir E., *Diabetes* 1965, 14:84.
19 ——Teitelbaum A., Balogh M., Groen J. J., *Amer. J. Clin. Nutr.* 1966, 19:59.
20 ——*Geriatrics* 1968, 23:158.
21 Doeblin T. D., Evans K., Ingall G., Frohman L. A., Bannerman R. M., *Diabetologia* 1969, 5:203.
22 Dohan F. C., Lukens F. D. W., *Endocrinol.* 1948, 42:244.
23 Duff G. L., Toreson W. E., *Endocrinol.* 1951, 48:298.
24 Ernest I., Linner E., Svanborg A., *Amer. J. Med.* 1965, 39:595.
25 Fabry P., Polidna R., Kazdova L., Braun T., *Nutritio et Dieta,* 1968, 10:81.
26 Gelfand M., Carr W. R., *Central Afr. J. Med.* 1961, 7:41.
27 Goldenberg S., Alex M., Blumenthal H. T., *Diabetes* 1958, 7:98.
28 Henry R. E., Burch T. A., Bennett P., Miller M., *Diabetes* 1969, 18:332.
29 Houssay B. A., Martinez C., *Science* 1947, 105:548.
30 Jackson W. P. U., *On Diabetes Mellitus,* Thomas Springfield, Illinois 1964, p.60.
31 Joslin E. P., Root W. F., White P., Marble A. *The Treatment of*

Diabetes, 10th ed. Lea and Febiger, Philadelphia 1959.
32 Kempner W., Peschel R. L., Schlayer C., *Post grad. Med.* 1958, 24:359.
33 Lacey P. E., *New Eng. J. Med.* 1967, 276:187.
34 *The Lancet* 1971, 1:381.
35 Lemonnier D., *Cahiers Nutr. Dietétique* 1967, 2:29 (*Nutr. Abst. Rev.* 2872:1968).
36 Macdonald I., *Amer. J. Clin. Nutr.* 1967, 20:345.
37 McGandy R. B., Hegsted D. M., Myers M. L., Stare F. J., *Amer. J. Clin. Nutr.* 1966, 18:237.
38 McKechnie J. K., *S. Afr. Med. J.* 1964, 38:182.
39 Miller M., Burch T. A., Bennett P. H., Steinberg A. G., *Diabetes* 1965, 14:439.
40 Mosinger B., Kujalora V., Lojda Z. 4th Congrès de la Fédération Internationale de Diabète. Editions Medicine et Hygiène Genève 1961.
41 Mouratoff G. J., Carroll N. V., Scott N. V., Scott E. M., *Diabetes* 1969, 18:29.
42 ——, ——, ——, *Jour. Amer. Med. Ass.* 1967, 199:107.
43 Muri J., *Acta Med. Scand.* 1954, 149:211.
44 *Nutrition Reviews* 1962, 20:192.
45 Office of Health Economics, *The Pattern of Diabetes*, O.H.E., London. 1964.
46 O'Sullivan J. B., in *Diabetes: Proc. of the 6th Congress of International Diabetes Federation* (ed. J. Ostman) p.696. Amsterdam 1969.
47 Perley M. J., Kipnis D. M., *J. Clin. Invest.* 1967, 46:1954.
48 Politzer W. M., Schneider T., *S. Afr. Med. J.* 1962, 36:608.
49 Prior I.A.M., Rose B. S., Harvey H. P. B., Davidson F., *The Lancet* 1966, 1:333.
50 Reid J. M., Fullmer S. D., Pettigrew K. D., Burch T. A., Bennett P. H., Miller M., Wheelon G. D., *Amer. J. Clin. Nutr.* 1971.
51 Schmidt-Nielsen K., Haines H. B., Hackel D. B., *Science* 1964, 143:689.
52 Seftel H. C., *S. Afr. Med. J.* 1961, 35:66.
53 Smith M., Levine R., *Med. Clin. N. America* 1964, 48:1387.
54 Sowton E., *Brit. Med. J.* 1962, 1:84.
55 Stein J. H., West K. M., Robey J. M., Tirador D. F., *Ann Intern. Med.* 1965, 116:842.
56 Toreson W. E., *Amer. J. Path.* 1951, 27:327.
57 Uram J. A., Friedman L., Kline O. L., *Amer. J. Physiol.* 1958, 192:521.
58 Von Noorden C., *Clinical Treatise on the Pathology and Therapy of Disorders of Metabolism and Nutrition*, New York E.B. Treat & Co. 1905 pt. VII.
59 ——*Klin Wchnschr* (Berlin) 1905, 36:817.
60 ——*Neuzeitliche Diabetesfragen*, Berlin and Vienna Urbau 1933.
61 West K. M., Kalbfleisch J. M., *Diabetes* 1970, 19:656.
62 Wilkerson H. L. C., Krall L. P., *J. Amer. Med. Ass.* 1947, 135:209.
63 Wood M. M., *Med. Proc.* 1960, 6:140.
64 Yudkin J., *Proc. Nutr. Soc.* 1964, 23: No. 2 149.

Thirteen

Peptic ulcer

Peptic ulcer in this context will refer predominantly to the disease of duodenal ulcer. Duodenal ulcer is more common than gastric ulcer in the countries of western civilisation at a ratio of 20:1.[36, 73] The conditions do however overlap.

Peptic ulcer is a disease with a strong hereditary influence. The leading aetiological factor in the environment is undoubtedly psychological stress with unwise nutrition and smoking of cigarettes playing subordinate roles. Its prevalence in western civilised countries has greatly increased over the last 60 years (Fig. 13.1),[72] though now showing signs of levelling out. Incidence of perforation of peptic ulcer, a surgical emergency leading to admission to hospital, has actually declined in certain areas of Britain since 1955.[54, 62] This fall however might merely indicate better preventive treatment from the general practitioner. From a general viewpoint peptic ulcer can be categorised as a disease of modern civilisation. The environmental factors causally related to it are peculiar to urbanisation in particular.

Pathogenesis of peptic ulcer
At the cellular level the development of a duodenal ulcer is dependent upon oversecretion of acid from the stomach,[3, 41] hypersecretion of the digestive enzyme pepsin and impairment of mucosal resistance.[51] The three factors no doubt vary in their proportionate role but the final common pathway of the disease almost certainly depends upon an oversecretion of acid and pepsin operating upon a decreased mucosal resistance. There have now been shown to be a number of clinical conditions, such as chronic lung disease and cirrhosis which predispose to peptic ulcer by the influencing of one

227

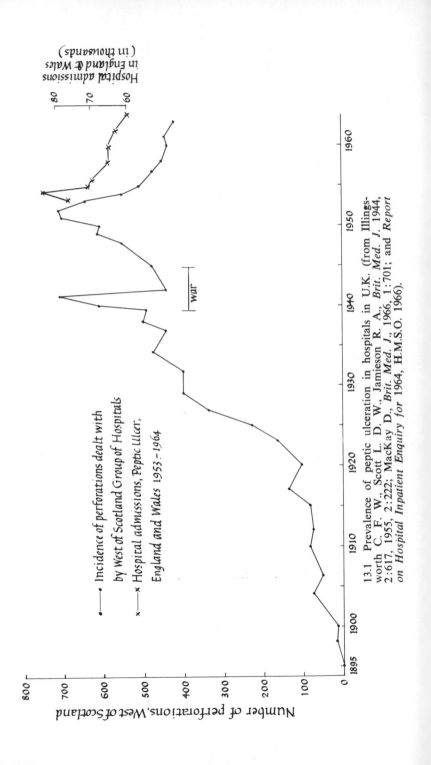

13.1 Prevalence of peptic ulceration in hospitals in U.K. (from Illingsworth C. F. W., Scott L. D. W., Jamieson R. A., *Brit. Med. J.* 1944, 2:617, 1955, 2:222; MacKay D., *Brit. Med. J.*, 1966, 1:701; and *Report on Hospital Inpatient Enquiry for 1964*, H.M.S.O. 1966).

Hospital admissions in England & Wales (in thousands)

Number of perforations, West of Scotland

• Incidence of perforations dealt with by West of Scotland Group of Hospitals

×—— Hospital admissions, Peptic Ulcer, England and Wales 1953 - 1964

war

of these three factors mentioned. There have also been shown to be a number of drugs that precipitate an ulcer either by stimulating acid production or by decreasing mucosal resistance, so highlighting the importance of these local factors.

Heredity

Two factors, parietal cell mass and Blood Group 0 are associated with peptic ulceration in man.[7] They both are associated with the hypersecretion of acid found in peptic ulcer subjects, and probably with factors such as mucosal resistance and antigen-antibody status of the mucosa, at the present time ill-understood. Peptic ulcer runs certainly in families[20, 66] and there is a high concordance rate in monozygotic twins.[25] Blood group 0 individuals are 40% more liable to peptic ulceration than members from other blood groups.[1] The absence of certain blood group antigens also correlates with the disease.[11]

Stress

Operating against this genetic background the dominant aetiological factor in the environment is almost certainly psychological stress. It has been conclusively shown that unpleasant emotional stimuli can establish a conditioned reflex that can result in continued abnormal gastric secretion.[6] The importance of such stimuli (e.g. tension at place of work, or in the home) has long been realised.

The now famous experiments conducted by Wolf and Wolff[77] on the exposed stomach of a certain patient showed how emotions could affect the state of the gastric mucosa. Fear and sadness evoked pallor of the mucous membrane and inhibition of gastric secretion. Anxiety and hostility on the other hand brought increased secretory activity, hypermotility and hyperemia of the gastric mucosa. Wolf and Glass[78] observed in a fistulous subject (where the stomach was exposed) that during sustained personal conflict with anxiety and resentment, gastric acid and gastric pepsin were increased. The concentration of muco-proteose (the secretion of the lining columnar epithelium) was low and under these circumstances the membrane was red and engorged and susceptible to injury.

In occupational surveys of peptic ulcer both foremen and executives have been shown to be peculiarly susceptible to the disease.[29, 35, 58] Both persons in their work face 'conflict' situations, where tension is likely to be created. In Scandinavian countries agricultural workers have lower peptic ulcer rates than their landowners.[2] Other surveys show rural workers to be less susceptible to the disease than city men[21, 53] Weir[74] notes the same phenomenon in Scotland. Doll et al.[21] reveal in their large survey on London that those who expressed anxiety over their work, such as foremen, were more likely to have a duodenal ulcer than other workers. High rates for duodenal ulcer have also been recorded in sea pilots who carry much executive responsibility. Among them the highest rates occur in those working the longest hours.[15] Not all executives however are prone to ulcer, and Weir[73] found a lower incidence in Scottish executives than expected. Others have found foremen prone but not executives.[24] The difficulty lies in measuring 'stress' against any human background. To a degree we are all affected by stress. Psychological factors were also thought to contribute to the rise in incidence of peptic ulcer noted at the start of the Second World War (see Fig. 13.1).[64, 68, 76]

In the experimental animal duodenal ulcers have been produced in monkeys.[9, 59] When placed in circumstances where one of a pair was obliged to assume 'executive responsibility' in the avoiding of electric shocks to itself and its companion the executive monkey developed duodenal ulcer (dying on occasions from perforation) while the passive member did not. An attempt by others however to reproduce this result failed.[27]

In an elegant study in Sweden carried out in 1968, Eberhard[25] examined 100 pairs of dissimilar and similar twins where proven peptic ulcer had occurred in the pair. Of the pairs examined 34 were monozygotic. Comparing those prone to ulcer in these twin studies against those not prone, it was revealed that ulcer individuals were more ambitious, and more tense than controls, more sensitive to criticism, moody and restless. It was summarised that they had an increased sensitivity to stress coupled with great ambitions. No indications appeared however of a specific personality type in the traditional sense, in contrast to the findings of certain psychoanalysts.[28, 79] On the other hand experimental evidence emerged in favour of the existence of psychological conflict internalised, as described some time ago by Alexander[15] (the struggle between internal parent and external authority with inability to release emotions in open aggression), and recently by others.[28, 80]

230

Smoking

Smoking has been correlated with peptic ulcer incidence[10, 22] as has also the drinking of alcohol.[31] Both might derive their connection with the disease from the personality type involved rather than by possessing primary causal properties. However the avoidance of smoking[23] definitely accelerates healing of an ulcer and smoking may have a physiological bearing upon ulcer formation. It is known to deplete the body of a certain amount of ascorbic acid and duodenal ulcer patients are known to be low in ascorbic acid.[26]

Diet and nutrition

Peptic ulcer shows interesting geographical variations in prevalence within a country and these cannot be ascribed to psychological factors. Peptic ulcer incidence is 15 times higher in South India for instance than in North India,[18, 30] varies considerably between South and North Nigeria,[16, 38] and is higher in North England and Scotland than in South England.[70, 71, 73] Malhotra[42] has correlated the distribution of the disease within India to the humidity and climate and hence to the type of food eaten. Others also[12, 50] have pointed out differences in diet between North and South India that could account for differences in disease incidence and some of these different dietary theories are reviewed here.

Epidemiologically speaking the most interesting country from an ulcer point of view is India. For some time now great differences have existed between South and North India as regards ulcer prevalence. The South Indian has always had a higher prevalence of the disease. This difference could be due to genetic factors. It could also be due to dietary differences. McCarrison[48] was one of the first workers to notice and work upon this difference. He noted that while the North Indian fed upon whole wheat chapattis, butter, plenty of vegetables, legumes, milk and some meat, the South Indian made do with rice, rice water, red pepper, tamarind (a spice) and a little fish, a much poorer diet deficient in certain of the vitamins A, B and C. The deficiency could have been the cause of the ulceration. Feeding these different diets to rats McCarrison[49] induced gastric ulcer in the poorly-fed 'South Indian' rats in 11% of cases and none in those fed whole wheat chapattis etc. Feeding the rats an even worse diet consisting of tapioca root, white rice and a little fish and red pepper, a diet current at the time amongst the people of Travancore in South India, McCarrison induced gastric ulceration in 28% of rats, but *not* duodenal ulceration.

Other workers had shown that vitamin deficiency can induce changes in gastric and duodenal mucosa[32, 34, 45, 47, 57, 61] but not specific duodenal ulceration,[19] and it is duodenal ulcers that out-number gastric ulcers by a ratio of 12:1 in Madras in McCarrison's time,[8] 36:1 in Travancore[65] and 20:1 in the West at the present time. If diet is to be implicated more subtle reasoning must be employed. Malhotra and Cleave have attempted this.

Malhotra[42] explains the high incidence of duodenal ulcer in South India also on the basis of diet but not by reason of malnutrition or vitamin deficiency. Malhotra's thesis rests upon the argument that different foods produce different quantities of saliva and saliva is a buffer to gastric acidity.[52] Fibrous foods are beneficial as they produce a thick saliva that buffers well. Sloppy foods such as tapioca, boiled rice and curry as eaten in South India produce little saliva and lead to greater gastric acidity. Hence the higher incidence of duodenal ulcer in the South. Malhotra[44] supports his thesis by showing that saliva from human volunteers chewing thick whole wheat diets has a higher buffering capacity than saliva produced by eating boiled rice diets. The theory needs more attention paid to it for its possibilities and research conducted to assess its validity outside India. Much of our food in the western world today is soft food and produces but little chewing or saliva. Is this a factor in ulcer production? The high incidence of ulceration in Scotland and North England compared to South England might be due to the higher consumption of refined carbohydrates in that area and lower consumption of fruit and vegetable (see Chapter 1).

Cleave[12, 13, 14] argues also for the refining of food and in particular, carbohydrates, as a principal cause for peptic ulceration. Cleave argues that protein buffers gastric acidity. Much of our food today has been refined and has had the protein 'stripped' from it as Cleave puts it. In this process principally in sugar and flour, protein is lost from the foodstuff and the concentrated carbohydrate content leads to high unbuffered gastric acidity in the stomach and duodenum. In the susceptible subject this predisposes to peptic ulceration. Cleave advances epidemiological evidence to show that peptic ulcer is a disease associated with peoples eating westernised foodstuffs. In contrast, where the diet becomes primitive and composed of unrefined foodstuffs, as in certain prisoner of war camps in the last war and within the German army on their Eastern front, peptic ulcer incidence drops.

Some confirmation is given to Cleave's hypothesis by Lennard Jones et al.[39] These workers showed that a high protein meal produced a smaller rise in acidity than a low protein meal, and that feeding maize cornflour produced a higher gastric acidity than feeding unrefined maize. But their results as regards bread carry less conviction. The protein content varies but little between wholemeal and white bread and by the Food Composition tables of McCance and Widdowson[46] the difference amounts to but 0.2%. Allinsons wholemeal bread contains 8.2% protein by weight while white bread contains 8.0%. One does not eat flour uncooked but even if one did the difference between wholemeal and white flour is again small. To achieve any difference in resulting gastric acidity in their experiments, Lennard Jones et al. had to especially enrich their brown bread with wheat germ, high in protein. A bigger difference exists between wholemeal and white bread as regards fibrous consistency and overall Malhotra's thesis is more convincing in this particular respect than Cleave's. Snacks quickly eaten, snatched between business engagements, bolted in half-hour lunch breaks, cannot do anybody's stomach much good, and add to the strain thrown upon our poor gastro-intestinal tract by the stress of modern living.

Where there is a theory regarding sugar there is one regarding fat, and a certain Jaques Spira[67] has contributed a monograph on the subject incriminating the consumption of fat in the Western world as the cause of peptic ulcer! He has given 4000 references or more to his work! His main contention being that fat raises and prolongs gastric acidity, exposing the duodenum to assault from the hyperacid juices. Further regurgitation of bile from the action of fat leads to gastro duodenal ulceration. Against this theory it must be remembered that milk and cream were at one time diets given *for* ulcer treatment, and that a country such as South India with a high incidence of duodenal ulcer has a low consumption of fat.

In summarising the place of nutrition in the causation of peptic ulcer, the author feels the following can be stated. Wholesome food· with a high content of roughage, with a fair quantity of fresh fruit and vegetable that has to be chewed and masticated thoroughly, eaten quietly and peacefully is ulcer-preventing. Café food and canteen snacks that are bolted, eaten in haste, and which are generally refined in quality needing little mastication, are ulcer-provoking.

Prevalence

Weir and Backett[75] show that in the North of Scotland in an urban community, 30% of the population suffer mild dyspepsia and indigestion at any one time, 15.4% severe dyspepsia and indigestion and 10.2% have a demonstrable peptic ulcer. Doll, Jones and Buckatzsch[21] find 6% of Londoners with actual ulceration and 10% of men between the ages of 45 and 54.

Morbidity from this condition is high. Five million working days are lost annually to this illness[37, 56] accounting for a loss of income of £12 million. Medical care for the disease costs in the neighbourhood of £7-8 million.[55]

Its incidence in the population has increased seemingly tenfold in this century[33] though indications are that the rise is levelling off and acute emergencies beginning to fall off.[33, 69] Most countries in Northern Europe report similar rises in incidence in this century[2, 4, 40, 63, 72] and Scotland has one of the highest death rates for peptic ulcer in Europe at 10 per 100,000. The most consistent correlation found associated with peptic ulcer in the West is urbanisation.[2, 21, 53, 60] In this chapter some of the reasons for this have been explored. It has been shown that while psychological stress is the dominant factor in aetiology, diet does play a role and that soft non-fibrous low protein, high carbohydrate foods could be culpable in this respect.

REFERENCES TO CHAPTER 13

1 Aird I., Bentall H. H., Mehigan M. B., Roberts J. A. F., *Brit. Med. J.* 1954, 2:315.
2 Alsted G., *The Incidence of Peptic Ulcer in Denmark,* Danish Science Press, Copenhagen 1953.
3 Atkinson M., Henley K. S., *Clin. Sci.* 1955, 14:1.
4 Bager B., *Acta Chir. Scand.* 1929, 64: Supp. 1.
5 Becker B. J. P., quoted by Straub M., Scharnagle H. E., *Schweiz Z., Path.* 1958, 21:250.
6 Bockus H. L., *Gastroenterology,* vol. 1. p.432. W. B. Saunders & Co., Philadelphia & London 1963.
7 ——*Gastroenterology,* vol. 1 p.446. W. B. Saunders & Co., Philadelphia & London 1963.

8 Bradfield E. W. C., *Transactions of the 77th Congress, Far Eastern Association of Tropical Medicine* 1927 Vol. 1, p.221. Thackers Press and Directories, Calcutta 1927.

9 Brady J. V., *Sci. Amer.* 1958, 199:95.

10 Brown R. G., McKeown T., Whitfield A. G. W., *Brit. J. Prev. Soc. Med.* 1959 13:131.

11 Clarke C. A., Edwards J. H., Haddock D. R. W., Howel Evans A. W., McConnell R. B. *Brit. Med. J.* 1956. 2:725.

12 Cleave T. L. *Peptic Ulcer*, Bristol, John Wright & Sons, 1962.

13 ——*Amer. J. Proctology* 1964 15:297.

14 ——Campbell G. D., *Diabetes, Coronary Thrombosis and the Saccharine Diseases*, Bristol, John Wright & Sons, 1969.

15 Dalhamm T., *Brit. J. Ind. Med.* 1953, 10:157.

16 Davies D. T., Wilson A. T. M., *The Lancet* 1939, 2:723.

17 Dogra J. R., *Ind. J. Med. Res.* 1940, 28:145.

18 ——*Ind. J. Med. Res.* 1940, 28:481.

19 ——*Ind. J. Med. Res.* 1941, 29:311.

20 Doll R., Buch J., *Ann Eugenics* 1950, 15:135.

21 ——Jones F. A., Buckatzsch M. M., *Med. Res. Coun. Spec. Rep.* Series No. 276, 1951.

22 ——Hill A. B., *Brit. Med. J.*, 1956, 2:1071.

23 ——Jones F. A., Pygott F., *The Lancet* 1958, 1:657.

24 Dunn J. P., Cobb S., *J. Occup. Med.* 1962, 4:343.

25 Eberhard G., 'Peptic ulcer in twins', *Acta Psych. Scand.* suppl. 205, 1968.

26 Esposito R., Valentine R., *Brit. Med. J.* 1968, 1:118.

27 Foltz E. I., Millett F. E., *J. Surg. Res.* 1964, 4:445.

28 Goldberg E. M. *Family Influences and Psychosomatic Illness.* Tavistock Press, Lond. 1958.

29 Gosling R. H., *J. Psychosom. Res.* 1957, 2:190.

30 Hadley G. G., *Ann Rep. Ind. Council Med. Res.* 1959, p.31.

31 Hagnell O., Wretmark G., *J. Psychosom. Res.* 1957, 2:35.

32 Hanke M., *Klin Wchnschr* 1937, 16:1205.

33 Illingworth C. F. W., Scott L. D. W., Jamieson R. A., *Brit. Med. J.* 1944, 2:617.

34 Ivy A. C., Grossman M. I., Barach W. H., Churchill, London. 1950. p.306.

35 Jacques E., *The Changing Culture of a Factory*, Dryden Press, N.Y. 1952.

36 Jamieson R. A., *Brit. Med. J.* 1955, 2:222.

37 Jones G. M., *Brit. J. Prev. Soc. Med.* 1959, 13:74.

38 Konstam P. G., *The Lancet* 1954, 2:1039.

39 Lennard Jones J. E., Fletcher J., Shaw D. G., *Gut* 1968, 9:177.

40 Levij I. S., *The Acute and Chronic Peptic Ulcer of Stomach and Duodenum*, Excelsior, The Hague, Holland 1959.

41 Littmann A., *Gastroenterol* 1962, 43:166.

42 Malhotra S. L., *Gut* 1964, 5:412.

43 —— Majumdar C. T., Bandoloi P. C., *Gut* 1964, 5:355.

44 ——Saigal O. N., Mody G. D., *Brit. Med. J.* 1965, 1:1220.

45 Manville I. A., *Amer. J. Physiol.* 1933, 70:105.

46 McCance R. A., Widdowson E. M., *Composition of Foods*, Med. Res. Counc. Spec. Rep. Ser. No. 297.

47 McCarrison R., *Ind. J. Med. Res.* 1919, 7:167.

235

48 ——*Brit. Med. J.* 1931, 1:1009.
49 ——*Ind. J. Med. Res.* 1931, 19:61.
50 ——*Brit. Med. J.* 1936, 2:611.
51 Menguy R., *Amer. J. Dig. Dis.* 1964, 9:199.
52 ——Masters Y. F., Gryboski W., *Surgery* 1965, 58:535.
53 Morris J. N., Titmuss R. M., *The Lancet* 19??, 2:841.
54 Morris J. N., *Uses of Epidemiology,* 2nd ed. Livingstone, Edinburgh, 1964.
55 Office of Health Economics, *Costs of Medical Care*, O.H.E., London 1964.
56 ——*Work Lost through Sickness,* O.H.E., London. 1965.
57 Orr I. M., Rao M. V. R., *Ind. J. Med. Res.* 1939, 27:159.
58 Pflanz M., Rosenstein E., Von Vexkull T., *J. Psychosom. Res.* 1956, 1:68.
59 Porter R. W., Brady J. V., Conrad D., Mason J. W., Galambos R., Rioch D. M., *Psychosom. Res.* 1958, 20:379.
60 Pulvertaft C. N., *Brit. J. Prev. Soc. Med.* 1959, 13:131.
61 Rao M. N., *Indian Med. Gaz.* 1943, 78:324.
62 Report of Hospital Inpatient Enquiry for year 1964, Hosp. Statistics Eng. and Wales PT.1 Tables 1964.
63 Romenius J., *Acta Med. Scand.* 1955. 152:391.
64 Short J. Rendle, *The Lancet* 1942, 1:429.
65 Somervell T. H., *Transactions of the 7th congress, Far Eastern Assoc. of Trop. Med.* 1927 Vol. 1, p.229, Thackers Press & Directories, Calcutta 1927.
66 Spiegel E., *Dt. Arch. Klin. Med.* 1918, 126:45.
67 Spira. J. Jaques, *Gastro Duodenal Ulcer,* Butterworth, London. 1956.
68 Stewart D. N., Winser D. M. de R., *The Lancet* 1942, 1:259.
69 Susser M., Stein Z., *The Lancet* 1962, 1:1115.
70 Watkinson G., *Gut* 1958, 1:4.
71 ——*Schweiz Z., Allg. Path.* 1958, 21:405.
72 ——*Gut* 1960, 1:14.
73 Weir R. D., *Scot Med. J.* 1960, 5:257.
74 Weir R. D., Brass W., *Brit. J. Prev. Soc. Med.* 1964, 18:102.
75 Weir R. D., Backett M., *Gut* 1968, 9:75.
76 Wilson A. K., *The Lancet* 1942, 1:335.
77 Wolf S. G., Wolff H. G. *Human Gastric Function, an Experimental Study of Man and his Stomach,* Oxford Univ. Press., London. 1947.
78 Wolf S., Glass G. B. S., *Fed. Proc.* 1950, 9:138.
79 Wretmark G., *Acta Psychiatr. Neurol. Scand.* 1953, *supp.* 84:1.
80 ——*J. Psychosomat. Res.* 1960, 5:21.

Fourteen

Sir Robert McCarrison and wholefood

To conclude the book on a positive note it is the aim of this last chapter to detail some of the evidence that shows how consumption of a good wholesome diet can promote true health of man, prevent disease and generally lead to a state of well being, surely the aim of any nutritionist, doctor or layman interested in diet, and the health of mankind.

Sir Robert McCarrison used to say that the greatest single factor in the acquisition and maintenance of good health was perfectly constituted food.[73] Such food was provided if three factors were satisfied:

(1) Food should be grown on a healthy soil.
(2) Food should be eaten whole.
(3) Food should be eaten fresh.

From his years studying nutrition in India and at home McCarrison[49, 50] stipulated the healthy ideal diet as that based on consumption of:

Wholegrain cereals
milk, milk products
legumes
fresh vegetables and fruit
(whilst meat was a luxury that could be eaten on occasions).

The three cornerstones of this diet are:

(1) healthy protein (from wholegrain cereals, pulses, milk);
(2) fresh vegetable;
(3) fruit.

This philosophy and understanding of nutrition is simple and sound enough to be taught anywhere in the world. Its message

237

could as well be applied by the housewife in London as the peasant in India. No need is there for explanation regarding carbohydrate, fat, calories, vitamin or mineral nutrition. The message of health is conveyed by emphasizing that these groups of foodstuff, good protein, fruit and raw vegetable, are the means to health, and the true base of a good diet.

· Sir Robert McCarrison was born in 1878 and died in 1960. He was famous for his pioneer work on vitamin nutrition in India, performed and carried out at the Research laboratories at Coonoor in the 1920s. Quick to observe that diets throughout India varied very much according to soil, climate and type of crop grown, he also observed that health and disease correlated with type of food eaten. The healthy Punjabis in North India ate wholewheat chapattis, milk, pulses (dhal) and vegetables while the unhealthy Madrassis in the South of India ate polished rice, some vegetables, dhal and coconut. McCarrison confirmed these observations in his laboratory by feeding these different diets to rats. The rats on the Punjabi diet throve while those on the Madrassi diet fell ill.[74]

Very importantly also McCarrison noted that vitamin deficiency could manifest in severe or chronic form. He pointed out that mild grades of deficiency were much more widespread amongst people than severe grades, and led as surely though more slowly to a lowering of vital processes, impaired resistance to microbic agents and development of diseases of many kinds. He pointed to the overconsumption of refined carbohydrates, white flour and sugar in the West as leading to diseases of lowered vitality and chronic nature and carried out experiments in rats to show the impairment to health of these foodstuffs. He stressed that abundance of food does not necessarily protect against food deficiency and outlined certain casualties of Western feeding. He pointed to the child of pale pasty complexion, unhealthy appetite and sluggish bowels, with mucus stools as one casualty. Another was the anemic adolescent with visceroptosis, acne or seborrhoea and vague psychological complaints, surviving on white bread, snacks and tea with sugar. Who does not recognize these sicknesses today as even then in McCarrison's time? Another case exampled was the exhausted and overstressed mother eating too little of the right food, existing on processed food, white flour, cups of tea and packaged conveniences of one sort and another, worried by dyspepsia to the point where she becomes actually unable to take any fresh vegetables at all.

The story is the same today but now, in view of the numbers involved and the changing nature of food, the problem assumes a national importance. McCarrison possessed a perception which was acute and in advance of his time, for he saw how chronic illness was linked to substandard nutrition and fed whole diets to his laboratory rats to prove his thesis. These experiments need repeating today and need to be adjusted to contemporary situations. For instance in one famous experiment McCarrison fed his rats a typical poor English diet of the time and compared the effect of this on the rats to a healthy Indian diet. The English diet consisted of white bread, vegetables cooked in water (à l'anglaise), margarine, tinned meat, tinned jam and sugar. The rats developed a craving for tea and sugar and consumed 600 ccs daily of this! The healthy diet on the other hand consisted of wholewheat flour, fresh vegetables, milk and pulses. The rats on an English diet had a mortality more than double that of those on a healthy diet and were ill-grown, poor-coated, weakly and listless. The results speak for themselves.

It has been the aim of this book to emphasise the conditions and illnesses that result from poor quality food eaten by a large proportion of the populace today. A few pilot experiments in the field have been carried out on communities to show the effect on health of reforming the diet along wholefood lines and these are outlined here in this chapter, for they provide interesting 'proof' of a kind. Also included in the chapter is a short account of the health of certain primitive communities and an analysis of the food these communities consume, for man can exist on a varied diet in many different situations and each situation can provide a lesson from which to learn. For primitive people the health-giving properties of a diet depend upon the balance of foodstuffs achieved (a balance which has evolved over thousands of years in these communities) and the natural unprocessed nature of the food. In some respects man's health is delicately poised in such situations and alteration and westernisation of a primitive diet can be disastrous. The final section of this chapter is given over to an analysis of certain protective and beneficial qualities possessed by raw vegetables, fruit and wholegrain cereals and the effect of these qualities on man. It *is* possible to formulate for man what might be truly termed a 'positively healthy diet.'

The food and health of western man
Wholefood diets
In the *Journal of the Soil Association,* over the years, a number of experiments have been recorded in which schools and institutions have been placed on wholefood diets and significant increase in health achieved by such means. Under the initiation of perhaps a general practitioner and controlled and assessed by such persons as a headmaster or a school matron, the surveys it will be seen are amateur, and open to observer bias, the uncontrolled variation of many factors and all the other pitfalls of such assessments, but for all this they provide interesting material for study. Alone, each survey is probably of little value. Together they mean more and may arouse enough interest to initiate a repetition of such experiments under more rigorous control.

Dr. G. B. Chapman, a general practitioner in New Zealand, was responsible for several of the studies here reported, which were carried out some 30 years ago on school populations in New Zealand. Chapman was interested to influence school and government authorities of his day with a view to the institution of dietary reforms amongst schools generally. Diets introduced under his supervision included such foods as wholemeal bread, honey, home grown and compost grown vegetables, salads, fruit and vitamin supplements. He was particularly keen that vegetables should be compost grown, and introduced this practice to the schools mentioned.

One of Chapman's first trials was carried out at the Mount Albert Grammar School in Auckland in 1936.[5] An account of this experiment was briefly written up in *Nature* in 1940.[17] The diet originally at the school had been 'liberal' but the boys nevertheless suffered frequent colds, catarrh, septic tonsils, flu and dental caries. In 1936 after an energetic campaign by Dr. Chapman the school put one acre of garden into compost production of vegetables and added to the diet a fair quantity of green vegetables, salads, pumpkins, root vegetables and fruit. Vitamin A and D supplements were also given. Matron three years later reports:

> During the past three years there has been a marked physical growth and development during heavy school work and sport . . . There are fewer accidents, particularly in the football season. . . . The first thing to be noted during the twelve months following the changeover to garden produce grown

from our humus treated soil, was the declining catarrhal condition among the boys. Catarrh had previously been general, and in some cases very bad among the boys. In specific cases the elimination was very marked and in many cases complete. There was also a very marked decline in colds and influenza. Colds are now rare and any cases of influenza very mild. During the 1938 measles epidemic, which was universal in New Zealand, the new boys suffered the more acute form of the attack; while the boys who had been at the hostel for a year or more sustained the milder attacks, with a much more rapid convalescence.

The matron also noted improved dental health and lack of gastric upsets. Dr. Chapman tried to interest the government at the time with the results claimed, without success.

A second experiment carried out by this doctor involved a school for 40 Maori children in Araminrio near Hamilton, New Zealand, in 1937.[39] The improved diet in this case covered but one meal a day, the midday meal. The garden as in the previous study was turned over to compost produce. Lunch consisted of soup, salad, whole wheat grains (steamed until tender)· cod liver oil and malted milk. The soup was particularly rich in meat, bones and vegetables an adequate lunch to say the least! Improvement was noted in skin disease (impetigo and scabies). Mental alertness was much improved among the 40 pupils, coughs and colds almost disappeared and a marked improvement in dental health took place (in 1940, 85% were free from decay).

A third experiment under Dr. Chapman took place about the same time in Manukau Intermediate School, Onehunga, Auckland.[40] 96 children were included in the experiment which this time included controls, half the children being fed the special lunch and half being given a standard lunch. The special lunch consisted of salad, cheese, fresh milk (with added skim milk powder and vitamins A and D), wholemeal bread and wheat germ. Colds were reduced by 34%. There was less fatigue, improved mental attention and increased participation in sport. Two physicians, a dental surgeon and others were brought in to assess improvement in the trial group. In this group there was 63% less dental decay, as compared to the control group, and cavities present were much smaller. Colds in the trial group lasted 75% shorter in time and school attendance records were improved.

A very similar trial to this was carried out about the same time in England at an L.C.C. School.[37] A special midday meal was introduced by the authorities at this school which meal consisted of wholemeal bread with butter, a raw vegetable salad of very varied content with grated cheese, half a pint of milk and half an apple at the finish. Again controls were provided in this experiment and results were as follows. An increase in height (70-100%) and weight (40-80%) of the trial group over the control was noted, a striking improvement in skin condition, improvement in nervous stability and mental capacity with enjoyment expressed by the children of their meal. The controls were fed a normal cooked lunch of meat, vegetables and pudding. Details are not given of calorie or vitamin values in any of these experiments.

A similar type of experiment to that of Dr. Chapman was carried out in America at North Country School, Lake Placid, New York State in 1950.[38] Inspired by Soil Association advice the headmaster of this school in that year turned his school vegetable garden over to organic methods of cultivation. Before doing so the garden had supplied much of the school vegetable produce for 10 years, being fertilised and sprayed in the conventional manner. During these years the garden had suffered much from drought and wind erosion. Then a change of policy was brought about and livestock were brought in to provide manure and compost, and in 1950 artificial fertilizers were discarded. Plants and vegetables apparently grew stronger from then on and the condition of the soil improved. Insect and disease infestation was thrown off by the healthy plants. No sprays or dusts were used from that period onwards.

Food from the garden was used daily in the school. Raw foods, especially green vegetables were served daily and included lettuce, endive, chicory and parsley in abundance. String beans, carrots, turnips, peas and cabbage were also often eaten raw! No sugar was allowed on the table, only 2 lb per person being used each year! Foods cooked were in the water for a minimum time and all cooking water was saved for gravies and soups.

Before these introductions to the dietary régime, health record at the school had been impressive, the children averaging five days illness per school year. Outdoor sports were encouraged, and a well balanced conventional diet was supplied with wholegrain cereals, vegetables, fruit included. After innovations mentioned, days illness per year dropped from 5 to 2 per child and a general measure of improved health was noted by the headmaster and others. Tooth decay decreased markedly. The headmaster noted in his account of the experiment how difficult health is to measure accurately but he nevertheless felt a significant change had taken place in the health of the school children and staff.

It is easy to criticize these experiments for, as explained in the introduction, the variable factors involved are many indeed. Dr. Chapman for instance added vitamin supplements or in some cases malted milk and cod liver oil to most of his reformed diets and almost certainly these changes alone produced some effect upon health. It is impossible in fact to emphasise one factor or group of factors as operative in improvements noted. However, important is the fact that general improvement in health occurred in these children, on broadly based dietary reforms. Comparing such diets to what is eaten nowadays by an average school child, the differences are extensive. Very few of our schools have their own vegetable gardens. Only one school in England is known to attempt composting. Soup in most schools is tinned not prepared from home produced vegetables. Salads are unpopular and consist of lettuce, cucumber and tomato, on the whole an unaesthetic combination if overdone! They tend therefore to be unpopular with children. Wholemeal bread, wheatgerm, vitamin supplements, malted milk, cod liver oil are on the whole not given. Milk has recently been curtailed in its supply to schools. The health of the schoolchild could be greatly improved if more enlightened attention was given to the problem of feeding than is evident today.

Wholefood diets and teeth

A wholefood diet would seem to affect incidence of tooth decay in children. Besides the results already recorded in the previous section a well controlled and accurately recorded trial was carried out by Lilienthal et al[45] and published in the *Medical Journal of Australia* for 1953. The study took place at Hopewood House Children's Home in New South Wales, Australia. 81 children were living in the home between the ages of four and nine. The survey carried out over five years was not controlled within the settlement but results were compared to controls provided by studies elsewhere in

New Zealand and Australia.

The experimental diet given consisted of wholemeal porridge, wholemeal bread, wheat germ, fresh and dried fruits, cooked and uncooked vegetables, butter, cheese, eggs, milk, fruit juices, vitamins, honey and nuts. Excluded from the diet were meat, sugar, white bread, white flour products and tea. Food was prepared as naturally as possible with the minimum of cooking.

The results showed a striking decrease in dental caries (see Table 14.1). A high degree of immunity from dental caries was found with a D.M.F. rate of 0.58 per child (5% of the New Zealand

TABLE 14.1

Dental health of children at Hopewood House as compared to dental health of children in other contemporary surveys

Site of Survey	Ages	Number of carious teeth per child d.m.f.	Percentage of children affected
Hopewood House	4 - 9	0.58	22
New Guinea 1950	6 - 10	2.7	60
Ontario 1951	5 - 9	8.0	92
Sydney 1953	4 - 9	9.57	96
New Zealand	7 - 9	11.38	95

Source: Lilienthal E. et al[45]

rate, 6% of the Sydney rate current at the time of the experiment). 63 children out of 81 remained free of caries for the 5 year period! The authors comment upon the small size of the lesions present, their slow initiation and slow growth, well below the rate found amongst the general population; and refer to an 'immunity' or 'resistance' against caries. Again it has not been the intention of the authors of this experiment to emphasise any one factor as important, rather to try to upgrade nutrition generally and observe results.

A similar investigation has been attempted more recently by Turner and Vickery[80] in Leicester. 103 children were investigated from families who followed 'wholefood' principles in their eating.

This was a loosely defined group but for the purposes of the experiment consisted of families that primarily ate 100% wholemeal bread in strict preference to white bread. Such families, it was noted, also restricted sugar intake and had a high consumption of fresh fruit and vegetables (raw and cooked). Inspection of the children's teeth showed (see Table 14.2) a D.M.F. rate of 2.0

TABLE 14.2

Dental health of children from wholefood families as compared to dental health of children from other contemporary surveys

Test Group	Age	Number of carious lesions per child d.m.f.	Percentage of children affected
Wholefood group	5	1.7	35
Northumberland			
Survey 1958	5	6.7	90
Seven counties			
Survey 1958	5	6.0	84
Wholefood group	6	2.5	58
Ministry of Health			
Survey 1961	6	6.2	91
Wholefood group	7	2.2	50
Ministry of Health			
Survey 1961	7	7.0	95

Source: Turner E., Vickery K.O.A.[80]   (where refs. are found to control material).

overall, compared to a national average of 5.8. Greatest differences existed at the age of 5, when an incidence of 1.7 D.M.F. amongst wholefood family children is compared to 6.5 and 7.0 amongst controls from other surveys. Gingival condition was counted very good amongst test subjects. Strict surveillance of diet was impossible under the circumstances but enough evidence is presented by these two surveys, that of Turner and Vickery and that conducted

245

by Lilienthal et al, to suggest that much dental caries, 50% and perhaps up to 80%, could be prevented by a wisely chosen diet.

Primitive races

Diets of primitive races though in the main far removed from that of our present day, are 'wholefood' in a sense, for they consist of food which is naturally grown, of an unsophisticated type and eaten raw. At that point the similarity is apt to finish. It is however instructive all the same to note the effect such diets have upon health and physique. Primitive peoples and races are often beset by various infective diseases, parasitic diseases and deficiency diseases if the local environment conduces to these. They are however strangely free of the so-called western diseases of civilisation. They suffer far less coronary heart disease, diabetes, peptic ulcer, rheumatism and arthritis, diverticulitis, dental caries, psychoneurosis, cancer of the lung etc. than is current in the West.

If survival against hazards of childbirth and infection is successful, longevity of age is not unknown in many instances and in the case of certain hill people and peasants in central Asia, life is often lived to a hundred years or more. Ages of up to 163 years[53] have been recorded.

Study of the diet of such people can contribute to our knowledge of the role that nutrition plays in health. But the contribution is a general one, for so many differences exist when the way of life of such people is compared to our own. It would therefore be unfair to pretend that any superiority in health was entirely due to diet, or one factor in the diet. The diet itself will differ in many respects to our own. Besides this the people in such areas do not experience the stress of urban living. They probably do not smoke cigarettes. They will take more exercise in living an outdoor peasant existence. Their genetic background will be totally different and their mineral intake will almost certainly vary substantially from ours. These are all factors that could contribute to differences in health. There are probably many others. It is thus probably true to say that the fact that they do not eat cornflakes, white sugar, eggs and bacon and coffee may be of secondary importance!

Sir Robert McCarrison[73, 74] in studying the natural diet of the different peoples in India before the last war was a pioneer in the world of nutritional epidemiological survey. McCarrison[51, 52] had observed that the physique, stature and health of the northern Indian was far superior to his brother in the South and that as one moved southwards through India a progressive deterioration in health occurred. Nutrition was an infant subject at the time and few studies accurately related diet to health in such a way as McCarrison attempted to achieve in India. In the north he observed that wheat was grown and the Punjabis, Sikhs, Baluchis and Rajputs from the north had good health. In the south more rice was grown, the Madrassis and Kanarese depending upon this as their main food. Their health was poor. Midway between the two extremes, the Maharatta combined both wheat and rice in their diet. The change from north to south was also accompanied by a change in amount of protein and vitamins consumed. Less milk and less wheat were consumed in the south and the diet there was of poor value. The strength of McCarrison's work lay in the fact that to prove the correlation between diet and health following these preliminary observations he carried out extensive feeding trials on rats. McCarrison fed diets identical to those eaten in various parts of India to groups of rats and observed their growth and health. The Sikh diet from the north consisted of freshly ground whole wheat (made into chapattis), milk, butter, curds, varied vegetable, tomatoes and fresh meat, with bone and fat once a week. The Madrassi diet from the south consisted of mashed polished rice, dhal, fresh vegetables, vegetable oil, coffee with sugar, a little milk, coconut and water. The Sikh rats grew well and strong to a final average body weight of 235 g. The Madrassi rats only grew to an average of 155 g. The intermediate Maharatta rats finished at 225 gms.

Convinced of the proven health of such a Sikh diet as outlined above, McCarrison maintained over 2,000 rats on this diet in his Coonoor laboratories over the years and recorded a remarkable degree of health amongst them.

Amongst health food folk lore, the Hunzas and stories about the Hunzas have for sometime occupied a special place. The land of Hunza lies in North West India, 8000 feet up in the Himalayas. Situated north westerly from Kashmir, Hunza lies some 177 miles from the Sinkiang border. The people of Hunza live a quiet peasant existence, and they are poor, as peasants usually are. Many of them own a plot of land and where crowding and overpopulation have occurred a certain amount of poverty exists and health sometimes suffers. Undoubtedly population expansion has occurred in Hunza, as elsewhere, and the health record of the country suffered accordingly of recent years. McCarrison visited the country in the 1920s and commented upon the remarkable physique of this people 'unsurpassed by any Indian race'.[48] He observed no evidence of peptic ulcer, appendicitis, colitis or any other alimentary disorder and attributed this to the healthy diet of the people.

The Hunza's food consists of wholemeal bread and chapatti (barley and millet is also grown), apricots (in abundance), yoghurt, cheese and vegetables, often eaten raw. The drinking water is glacial in origin and carries a high silt content rich in various minerals. The Hunzas possess a record of longevity and bear towards life an easy going and relaxed attitude of which one might well be envious.

However recent appraisals[15, 54] of the health of this people show them to be not entirely clear of disease, indeed it would be remarkable if they were. Western civilisation has encroached upon this peaceful land and tinned foods, imported sugar and other benefits from the West have made impact upon the country's nutrition. Hunzaland is hardly therefore a Utopia. However the extent to which conditions have deteriorated over some 30 years is hard to assess and there is still a large measure of health amongst the old people as shown by the recent research of two cardiologists.

E. C. Toomey and Paul White[79], two cardiologists, recently travelled to Hunza and examined 25 aged Hunzas between 90 and 100 years old, for cardiovascular symptoms. They found none. The blood pressure of the group ranged from 120/70 to 150/90, and the cholesterol readings ran from 150 to 180 mg/100 ml, figures well below comparable western data. Electro-cardiographs taken, showed no evidence of heart disease. Toomey and White commented upon the spartan diet of these people which consisted of fruit, nuts, vegetables and grains (wheat, barley and millet), and upon the lack of observable disease in this group. In one area of health therefore the record of this group is untarnished.

Another primitive race studied that showed absence of heart disease and very low cholesterol readings was the group of Brazilian Indians studied by Pazzanese et al. in 1964.[57] These people ate fish, insects, larvae, corn, manioc, peanuts and sweet potatoes and the latter four items were often eaten raw. Honey, sugar cane,

248

bananas and fruits made up the diet. The diet contained no milk or meat, other than fish and was therefore exceptionally low in fats. What fats are eaten were mostly unsaturated. The blood lipid and cholesterol fractions were very low compared to American standards, and there was little evidence of arteriosclerosis.

The Bantu[82] in South Africa are another race that have been studied in an attempt at clear understanding of relationships between diet and heart disease. The food of the Bantu in the rural areas, consists of maize, wheat, kaffir corn (sorghum) and small amounts of legume vegetables (cow peas and sugar beans). The diet is high in fibre and low in fat. The Bantu, similarly to the Brazilian Indians record a low cholesterol count and low incidence of heart disease.[9] Walker[83] rightly points out the difficulty of interpreting such data when many other factors besides diet are known to affect heart disease.

Eskimoes[65] have also been studied, and have held interest for nutritionists for the high meat and fat diet they consume. However in contrast to the West the meat is often raw and fat is of an unsaturated type. The primitive Eskimo, the hunter, lives off fish, seal meat and caribou, partly eaten raw and eaten together with a few berries and edible plants. The small proportion of vegetable foods is compensated for by consumption of the stomach contents of fresh game. A large amount of berries are collected in the short summer and in June and July the leaves of tundra herbs are collected and eaten. Fresh meat can also contain a small amount of vitamin C. Schaefer[65] comments on the rarity of vitamin and mineral deficiences amongst the true primitive Eskimo, while heart disease is unknown under the age of 60, and of a lesser frequency over this age than is found in America. No case of peptic ulcer was recorded by Schaefer. Diabetes mellitus was very rare as was also dental caries.

Unfortunately such races as the North Indian and Eskimo, as well as many other primitive peoples, suffer a certain susceptibility to modern degenerative disease and vitamin deficiency when they encounter modern food stuffs. The delicate balance of a naturally evolved nutrition and racial culture is all too easily upset by encounter with modern commercial foods. Each primitive race has developed a diet that achieves health, and often optimum health, within an ecological setting. Man's adaptability enables this to take place. Cheap, attractive and accessible imports of sugar, flour, and tinned foodstuffs take away the drive and initiative that were originally necessary in the hunt for food. Lax habits develop and ignorance contributes to a decay in nutritional standards and disease quickly follows. This has been recorded in the Eskimo and the North Indian and many other races. It is perhaps understandable but nevertheless regrettable. Dr. Mary Jackson[36] records this sequence well in the history of the North Indian in America and Schaefer[65] shows how the Eskimo is also corruptible.

Protective factors in wholefood diets

It has been shown that there are certain factors in wholegrain cereals, fruit and raw vegetable that promote health. The first and obvious factor in fruit and vegetable is vitamin C.

Szent Gyorgyi first isolated ascorbic acid from the adrenal cortex in 1928. The main property of the substance is that of a reducing agent and the vitamin is used in many biological oxidation reactions within the body. Cellular respiration cycles are examples of these. Ascorbic acid is also used in the formation of collagen in connective tissue, the laying down of bone matrix, the metabolism of carbohydrate, the chemical inter-relationship betwen insulin and mineralocorticoids, the formation of adrenal cortical hormones and many other reactions.[1, 14, 58]

The vitamin is intimately associated with the body's metabolic reactions to stress. Trauma, fractures, burns, tissue injury, and infections deplete the body of vitamin C[2, 10, 24, 46] and Harris et al.[33] show how an injection of diphtheria toxin in guinea pigs depletes the adrenal gland of vitamin C. Cold exposure, anoxia and haemorrhage are other conditions where vitamin C is lost from the body. It is not surprising therefore to find, following this, evidence that vitamin C can protect the body against stresses of this nature. In guinea pigs the resistance and adaptation of the animal to a cold environment depends upon amount of C ingested daily.[21] Mice too depend on the vitamin in the cold.[9] Cats survived longer after acute haemorrhage with the aid of vitamin C[77] and guinea pigs, rats and mice benefited from the vitamin when sustaining trauma and shock.[81] The effect of burns however has not been shown to be lessened by C administration[4] and prophylactic effects generally in man have been slow to show as evidence.[27] Holmes[35] claimed that the vitamin prevented some of the effects

250

of physical trauma in man.

In medical treatments vitamin C has been shown to be an important requirement for wound healing.[59] It has been shown to improve periodontal health markedly and prevent gingivitis.[23] A study carried out by the Food Education Society (160 Piccadilly, London, W.1) and published in 1969 showed the effect of 50 mg vitamin C *given as fresh orange juice* in the prevention of coughs and colds. Two schools and two factories were involved in the double blind trial and incidence of colds was reduced markedly in the trial group.

Vegetables are rich in minerals, trace elements, chlorophyll and vitamin C. They also contain vitamins B1 and B2, carotene, vitamin K, cellulose· organic acids (tartaric, citric, malic etc.) small quantities of albumin, carbohydrates and bioflavinoids. Green vegetables contain a surprising amount of vitamin B1 and B2. Green peas for instance contain 0.30 mg of B1 per 100 g of edible portion, carrots 0.18 mg and spinach 0.16 mg. Spinach contains 0.23 mg of B2 per 100 g of edible portion and peas 0.16 mg. Fresh vegetables are nearly all important sources of carotene. Spinach, red pepper, lettuce, carrots, green pepper, cress, tomato are all rich sources of this vitamin precursor. Fresh vegetables are very rich in potassium salts as against sodium and are relatively rich in calcium. Cauliflower, beet, turnip, swede, cabbage all contain calcium in amounts ranging from 60 mg per 100 g in the case of cabbage to 200 mg per 100 g in the case of water cress. Iron, copper and iodine are constant components of vegetables.

Fruits are similarly rich in vitamins and mineral substances and constitute a nutritious food in themselves. It is a mistake to regard them as an inessential luxury. Citrus fruit is acknowledged as the richest available source of vitamin C but in addition contains vitamins of the B group and vitamin P (bioflavinoids). Half a grapefruit contains 35 mg vitamin C, 0.2 mg niacin, 1.4 mg pantothenic acid, 0.05 mg folic acid and small amounts of many other B vitamins. Fruit is also an important complementary source of calcium, iron and copper. It has been said that the citric acid in fruit aids the retention of calcium in the body and it has also been shown that orange juice aids the absorption of iron from such sources as bread.[12] Citric acid, malic acid and tartaric acids in fruit, following their metabolism within the body, form an alkaline urine and are thus less drain upon the alkaline reserves of the body. All these are advantages in maintaining health.

One of the most interesting components of fruits, and to a lesser extent vegetables, is vitamin P. Known today under the generic term 'bioflavinoids',[11] these substances are yellow pigments extensively distributed in fruit and green leaves. Particularly high concentrations are found in blackcurrants, rosehips and citrus fruit. Rutin, hesperidin and quercitin have been the most extensively studied. A chemical derivative of these compounds (chalcone) acts like ascorbic acid as a reducing agent in the body. The bioflavinoids have been shown to decrease capillary permeability and fragility. They have also been shown to partially inhibit tissue inflammatory response, and have been used in the treatment of varicose disorders, haemorrhoids and diabetic retinitis where capillary permeability is affected and tissue inflammation found. Fitzgerald[26] in a well conducted double blind trial found that injected bioflavinoids significantly improved varicose disorders in the leg and others have reported improvement in varicose vein conditions.[22] Benefit has also been found in haemorrhoid treatment.[7] Bleeding, severe pain and pruritus were all improved by bioflavinoids.[16] Sokoloff[76] showed they were effective in preventing x-ray radiation erythema by virtue of their effect upon capillary permeability. Rutin has been claimed as effective in the prevention of vascular haemorrhage in hypertension.[71]

Another pharmacological component of fruits and vegetables that has relevance with regard to the treatment of modern diseases is pectin. Pectin is a carbohydrate found in the skins of many citrus fruits, and ordinary fruits as in the apple, and also in vegetables and sunflower seeds. It may constitute up to 1% of the fruit and has been shown to be effective in lowering blood cholesterol. Palmer and Dixon[56] carried out an experiment on sixteen volunteers who on a normal diet with an addition of pectin experienced lowering of serum cholesterol levels from 230 mg per 100 ml to 192 mg. Keys[41] had noted this effect earlier in his experiments on vegetable diets.

Vegetarian diets lower cholesterol levels in man. This has now been shown by several investigations. In 1952 Groen et al.[28] showed that pure plant diets caused a fall in serum cholesterol and Hardinge and Stare[29] carried out a study comparing cholesterol readings between a vegan group (strict vegetarians who do not eat milk, egg or cheese) a lacto-ovo-vegetarian group and a meat eating group. They found significantly lower cholesterol readings in the vegan group. Shaper and Jones[72] carried out a similar study with corresponding results. Possible causes for the lowered cholesterol reading found in vegetarians and vegans could be the lowered intake of saturated fatty acids, or the higher intake of pectin and fibre. Harding et al[30] found vegans took in 20-23 g of fibre a day, vegetarians 12-16 g a day and non-vegetarians 8-10 g a day. The effect of fibre ingestion on flora of the intestine was postulated as a reason for lowered cholesterol. Pectin also interacts upon bowel flora and may contribute to lowered serum cholesterol by this means. West and Hays[84] in a study of Seventh Day Adventists found that the vegetarians had lowered cholesterol readings compared to the meat eaters and had a higher consumption of fruits, vegetable and vegetable protein. Consumption of unsaturated fatty acids was similar in groups studied and could not therefore be the cause of cholesterol differences in this experiment. Factor or factors in fruit and vegetable were more likely the cause of these differences.

Dr. D. C. Hare,[31] of the Royal Free Hospital in 1936 carried out some interesting studies on the effect of a fruit and raw vegetable diet upon arthritis. The cases selected were ten in number and varied in clinical presentation. They included osteoarthritis, acute rheumatoid arthritis, chronic rheumatoid arthritis and 'muscular rheumatism'. The Bircher-Benner diet given consisted of oats muesli for breakfast with raw fruit, a raw vegetable salad for lunch of varied substance and a raw vegetable salad at night. Dried fruits such as apricot, and raisins were included along with nuts and 2 oz olive oil for salad dressing. The diet made up to 2000 calories consisted of 145 g carbohydrate, 35 g protein and 143 g fat. 3 oz of cream was allowed in the muesli which would account for the surprisingly high fat content of the diet. One pint of milk was also taken. Most naturopaths would decrease the amount of fat taken by eliminating cream and cutting down the amount of milk consumed. Dr. Hare kept her patients on this strict diet for two weeks and then added eggs, cheese and meat to modify the diet and raise the protein content, still however maintaining the large amount of vegetable and fruit consumed. Results were encouraging in that of the 12 cases, 8 definitely improved over a period of one to four weeks. Most marked was the relief of pain, muscular pain, effusion and stiffness in all patients. Hare queries whether this improvement was due to the low salt content of the diet. 2 cases improved up to the fifth week of the trial but relapsed on the modified diet, and 2 cases of longstanding rheumatoid arthritis underwent no change. One patient completely immobilized by rheumatoid arthritis of recent origin was improved after a month to the extent of being able to stand and walk without help. Conditions that improved most strikingly were those involving muscular rheumatism and synovitis of a non specific type.

Hare and Pillman-Williams[32] later repeated the trial on six patients with rheumatoid arthritis and noted again marked clinical improvement in five out of the six cases, the sixth absconding from the régime. Most of these patients in the second trial were under nourished and showed low vitamin C levels at the start of the trial. Vitamin C was added along with the Bircher-Benner diet, and high ascorbic acid levels noted throughout the trial.

Dr. Kuratsune[43] at the University of Kyushu in Japan, carried out an experiment on himself and his wife whereby a diet of 150 g of raw whole rice, ground and kneaded with water was taken with 500 to 1000 g of raw vegetables (carrots, turnips, radishes, cabbage, spinach etc.) and a little fruit. Calorie content of the food was estimated at 800-1040 calories, 28 g protein, 200 g carbohydrate, and 8 g of fat. Fine health was maintained on this diet over months. Following this for a period of sixteen days all the vegetables and the rice were cooked. Symptoms of oedema appeared and blood haemoglobin dropped. On returning to the raw vegetable diet symptoms disappeared and health was restored.

An experiment carried out under more exacting conditions was performed by Carlson and Froberg[13] on 12 men in Sweden recently. Investigating the effect of near fasting conditions and the sole consumption of vegetable and fruit juices upon blood lipids during severe exercise, 12 men were asked to walk 500 km over 10 days, taking no solid food. The men, aged 20-50 years old, walked 50 km per day and took during the day bottled mineral water (average consumption 3,200 ml), 30 ml of commercially bottled apple juice, orange and grape juice (5-60 calories) and 200 ml of freshly prepared carrot and red beet juice (60-80 calories). In the evenings 500 ml of canned bouillon soup was taken (200 calories). Vitamin and mineral tablets were taken. Total calorie intake was therefore 340 calories! The men retained very good health during the walk, apart from some tenosynovitis,

254

Sir Robert McCarrison and wholefood

blisters and red feet from the effect of walking. Cholesterol, triglyceride and lipid levels in the blood decreased markedly. Blood glucose levels dropped slightly in the first six days, then thereafter increased. All subjects lost weight (av. 6.9 kg) as might be expected. However, more remarkable was the degree of health achieved despite the undertaking of severe exercise on such a very low calorie intake. The nutrients supplied by the raw vegetable and fruit juices were obviously fully adequate to meet most of the demands of the body in such circumstances.

Yoghurt is often included in a wholefood diet and is claimed to give certain benefits to health. Natural yoghurt is made by fermenting milk with a culture of lactobacillus acidophilus, lactobacillus bulgaricus and streptococcus thermophilus. The milk if left 24 hours to ferment forms a thick acidified curd which is yoghurt. However such a 'fresh' and active compound is difficult to market as it is likely to continue fermenting if held in the shop too long, and hence the various brands of bland commercial yoghurt that have appeared in recent years.

The eating of yoghurt alters the intestinal flora of the subject producing a predominance of lactobacilli in the large gut.[68, 75] In vitro studies of some of the metabolites of lactobacilli show that these possess an antagonistic effect on many organisms including E. coli, Shigella and Salmonella.[47] This antibacterial action has been demonstrated by Seneca et al.[69] while A. H. and C. A. Bryan in a paper that appeared in *Drug and Cosmetic Industry* (March 1959)[19] report the inhibition of growth in Proteus colonies in the presence of lactobacilli and confirm that salmonella and shigella are prevented from multiplication, in the presence of lactobacilli. Danon et al.[18] found that E. coli if grown in yoghurt lost its viability in several hours and with pigs demonstrated that coliform bacteria were eliminated from the intestinal tract by the feeding of yoghurt. It has been shown also to destroy M. tuberculosis within 8 hours.[78]

This antibacterial action of yoghurt explains the success that has followed its institution as an antidiarrhoeal agent in paediatric medicine. A number of reports now exist to show that yoghurt possesses a curative effect in infantile diarrhoea. Beck and Neycheles[6] for instance in 59 cases that included 22 cases of antibiotic diarrhoea, 19 cases of epidemic diarrhoea and others, produced excellent results in 90% of subjects just by the feeding of

255

capsules of dried lactobacilli. Failures occurred in a few chronic cases of colostomy diarrhoea. Niv et al.[55] in a controlled American study on 45 infants under one year old who presented with severe diarrhoea, showed a superiority of treatment for yoghurt over neomycin. The yoghurt group recovered quicker taking an average of 2.76 days to regain normality of bowel function, the neomycin group taking 4.8 days. Rectal swabs on the infants were predominantly gram negative on admission. On discharge 65% of those on yoghurt treatment had gram positive stools, 35% of the neomycin group. The yoghurt administered in this case was analysed as containing:

Butterfat	1.6%
Casein	3.9%
Lactalbumin	0.9%
Lactoglobulin	0.1%
Lactose	6.9%
Lactobacilli bulgaricus	125 million/ml
Streptococci thermophilus	125 million/ml
Lactic acid	1%

A study in a Canadian hospital[44] showed that yoghurt fed to infants could prevent spread of epidemic diarrhoea. Raffle[61] in this country reports similarly good results in gastro-enteritis. Constipation too is helped by yoghurt. Ferrer and Boyd[25] gave a mixture of yoghurt and prune whip to 194 patients suffering from constipation of average age 71 years, a large number of whom were diabetic. Not only did bowel action improve but also the condition of the skin. Seborrhoeic dermatitis cleared, chronic diabetic ulcers healed and morale improved!

Full understanding of the changes that occur in the bowel microflora of man following upon the ingestion of different foods and of yoghurt is not available to us at the present time. Dubos and Schaedler[20] working upon mice showed that if the bowel flora could be maintained with a dominant balance of lactobacilli,

256

resistance against certain diseases and growth rate was improved. They showed that the integrity and health of the large bowel wall depended upon the presence of microflora in the gut. Seneca et al.[70] show that endotoxins from bacteria can be absorbed by the intestinal mucosa carried by the lymphatic system into the blood stream and cause systemic illness, the presence of lactobacilli in the gut militating against this. Post irradiation bacteremia most often involves infection from coliform organisms, the effect of irradiation being to break down resistance of the bowel wall.[42]

Certain foods such as meat, casein and other proteins cause an increase in coliform organisms[60] in the gut while lactose and cereals encourage the growth of lactobacilli.[42, 75] The flora of the large bowel may play a significant part in the pathogenesis of other diseases besides diarrhoea. Ask-Upmark[3] from Sweden in a letter to *The Lancet* describes how the giving of Lactobacillus acidophilus by mouth aided and greatly improved migraine in 8 out of 10 patients so treated. Read et al.[63] have described the remarkable effect L. acidophilus can have in hepatic encephalopathy as also have Rafsky et al.[62] Yoghurt and culture of the human colon with lactobacillus can obviously affect the health of the whole man and be of use in the treatment of systemic illness.

There are probably many unidentified factors in food that confer resistance and even possibly immunity in disease, which await eventual discovery. Experiments conducted by Schneider[66, 67] give evidence of the presence of some of these factors in wholewheat which in turn may explain the confusing differences that have been shown to exist between various diets. Schneider identified factors associated with bacterial contamination of wholewheat that gave resistance to mice against salmonella infection. He named these factors pacifarins. These are factors that exist on wholewheat created by an interaction between the wheat husk and aerobacter bacteria. Wholewheat in the natural diets fed to certain mice gave an added resistance to salmonella typhimurium. However as Schneider painstakingly points out conditions have to be set exactly right before resistance manifests. Only a certain mixture of virulent and avirulent challenging organisms and only a certain strain of hybrid mice showed the effect. Other pure strains of mice challenged with unmixed organisms gave no effect. This experiment emphasises the variability of the total environmental effect and how it is impossible to jump straight to easy conclusions.

257

The two diets, as operated by Schneider are set out below:

Natural diet		*Synthetic diet*	
Ground whole wheat	66 g	Casein	18 g
Dried whole milk	33 g	Glucose	72.5 g
Salt	1 g	Salts	4 g
		L-cystine	0.2 g
		Vitamins	5.25 g

The factor identified by Schneider was destroyed in milling and found to be missing from refined flour but was present in such diverse sources as malted barley, sprouts, dried green and black tea. When isolated finally it was found to be extremely potent, raising survival rates of mice from 10% to 90% in certain experiments.

Summary

It has been the aim of this book to bring together evidence to show that the way we eat produces many of the diseases we suffer from. In certain important areas, our health is deteriorating as is our nutrition. Remedies could be found and dietary advice given.

It has been the aim of this chapter to show that a healthy diet as formulated by Sir Robert McCarrison leads to positive health within the human being. It is stated by many that there is no evidence. This book has been written to show that there is evidence and plenty of it. It merely requires that we look at the evidence. Only by this means can the burden of chronic ill-health throughout this country and the western world begin to be lifted.

REFERENCES TO CHAPTER 14

1 Allegretti N., Vukadinovic G., Rahadjya L., *Amer. J. Physiol.* 1954, 177:264, 1955, 180:508.
2 Andreae U. A., Browne J. S. L., *Can. Med. Ass. J.* 1946, 55:425.
3 Ask-Upmark E., *The Lancet* 1966, 2:446.
4 Bacchus H., Toompas C. A., *Science* 1951, 113:1269.
5 Balfour E. B., *The Living Soil* 8th ed., Faber, London. 1948.
6 Beck C., Necheles H., *Amer. J. Gastroent.* 1961, 35:522.
7 Berson I., *Med. Hyg.* 1957, 15:168.
8 Bircher R., *Hunsa, das Volk das keine Krankheit Kennt*, 5th ed. Verlag Haus Huber, Bern 1956.
9 Booker W. M., De Costa F. M., Tureman J. R., Froix C., Jones W., *Endocrinol.* 1955, 56:413.

10 Bly C. G., Johnson R. E., Kark P. M., Consolazio C. F., *U.S. Armed Forces Med. J.* 1950, 1:615.
11 *Brit. Med. J.* 1969, 1:235.
12 Callender S. T., Warren G. T., *Amer. J. Clin. Nutr.* 1968, 21:1170.
13 Carlson L. A., Froberg S. O., *Metabolism* 1967, 16:624.
14 Chalopin H., Monton M., Ratsimamanga A. R., *World Rev. Nutr. Dietet.* 1966, 6:165.
15 Clark J., *Hunza, Lost Kingdom of the Himalayas*, Hutchinson, London. 1957.
16 Clyne M. B., Freeling P., Ginsborg S., *Practitioner* 1967, 198:420.
17 Daldy Y., *Nature* 1940, 145:905.
18 Danon S., Zhekov S., Kozareva M., *C. R. Acad. Bulgar Sci.* 1960, 13:749.
19 *Drug and Cosmetic Industry*, March 1959.
20 Dubos R., Schaedler R. W., *J. Expl. Med.* 1962, 115:1161.
21 Dugal L. P., Therien M., *Can. J. Med. Res.* 1947, 25:111.
22 Fabre J., Rudhardt M., *Med. Hyg.* 1962, 20:161.
23 Eb. Ashiry G. M., Ringsdorf W. M., Cheraskin E., *J. Periodont.* 1964, 35:251.
24 Faulkner J. M., Taylor F. H. L. *Ann. Intern. Med.* 1937, 10:1867.
25 Ferrer F. P., Boyd L. J., *Amer. J. Dig. Dis.* 1955, 22:272.
26 Fitzgerald D. D., *Practitioner* 1967, 198:406.
27 Glickman N. R., Keeton N., Mitchell H. H., Fahnestock M. K., *Amer. J. Physiol.*, 1946, 146:538.
28 Groen J., Tijong B. K., Kamminga C. E., Willbrands A. F., *Chem. Abst.* 1953, 47:4973g. (Voeding 1952, 13:556).
29 Hardinge M. G., Stare F. J., *Amer. J. Clin. Nutr.* 1954, 2:73.
30 ——Chambers A. C., Crooks H., Stare F. J., *Amer. J. Clin. Nutr.* 1958, 6:523.
31 Hare D. C., *Proc. Roy. Soc. Med.* 1936, 30:1.
32 ——Pillman Williams E. C., *The Lancet* 1938, 1:20.
33 Harris L. J., Passmore R., Pagel W., *The Lancet* 1937, 2:183.
34 Higginson J., Pepler W. J., *J. Clin. Invest.* 1954, 33:1366.
35 Holmes H. N., *Ohio State Med. J.* 1946, 42:1261.
36 Jackson M. P., *Journal of the Soil Assoc.* 1961, vol. 11, Oct. p.867.
37 *Journal of the Soil Assoc.* Jan. 1952, p.55.
38 ——Jan. 1958, p. 25.
39 ——July 1960, p.284.
40 ——October 1963, p.784.
41 Keys A., Anderson J. T., Grande F., *J. Nutr.* 1960, 70:257.
42 Klainer A. S., Gorbach S., Weinstein L., *J. Bact.* 1967, 94:383.
43 Kuratsune M., *Kyushu Memoirs of Med. Sciences* 1951 June 2/1-2.
44 La Rue A., *Can. Med. Ass. J.* 1960, 83:1002.
45 Lilienthal B., Goldsworthy N. E., Sullivan H. R., Cameron D. A., *Med. J. Aust.* 1953, 1:878.
46 Lund C. C., Levenson S. M., Green R. W., Page R. W., Robinson P. E., *Arch. Surg.* 1947, 55:557.
47 Mayer J. B., *Rep. Xth Int. Congress of Pediatrics*, Lisbon 1962.
48 McCarrison R., *'Studies in Deficiency Disease'*, Oxford Medical Press 1921.
49 ——*Brit. Med. J.* 1926, 2:730.
50 ——*Indian J. Med. Res.* 1927, 14:649.
51 ——*Brit. Med. J.* 1931, 1:1130.

52 ——*Indian J. Med. Res.* 1931, 19:61.
53 *Medical News* June 7th 1968 p.7.
54 Mons, Barbara, *High Road to Hunza* Faber, London 1958.
55 Niv. M., Levy W., Greenstein N., *Clin Pediatr.* 1963, 2:407.
56 Palmer G. H., Dixon D. G., *Amer. J. Clin. Nutr.* 1966, 18:437.
57 Pazzanese D., Portugal O. P., Ramos O. L., Finatti A. A. C., Lanfranchi W., Barreto H., *The Lancet* 1964, 2:615.
58 Pirani C. L., *Metabolism* 1952, 1:197.
59 ——Levenson S. M., *Proc. Soc. Exp. Biol. Med.* 1953, 82:95.
60 Porter J. R., Rettger L. F., *J. Infect. Dis.* 1940, 66:104.
61 Raffle E. J., *The Lancet* 1956, 2:1106.
62 Refsky H., Rafsky J. C., *Amer. J. Gastroent.* N.Y., 1953, 24:87.
63 Read A. E., McCarthy C. F., Heatin K. W., Laidlaw J., *Brit. Med. J.* 1966, 1:1267.
64 Rodale J. I., *The Healthy Hunzas,* Rodale Press, Emmaus, Pa., U.S.A. 1949.
65 Schaefer O. *J. Can. Med. Ass.* 1959, 81:248, 386.
66 Schneider H. A., *Science* 1967, 158:597.
67 ——*Proc. Nutr. Soc.* 1967, 26:1, 73.
68 Schroeder K., *Nord Med.* 1946, 30:935.
69 Seneca H., Henderson E., Collins A. *Amer. Pract. Digest. Treat.* 1950, 1:1252.
70 ——Lattimer J. D., Peer P., *J. Urol.* 1964, 92:603.
71 Shanno K. L., *Amer. J. Med. Sci.* 1946, 211:539.
72 Shaper A. G., Jones K. W. *The Lancet* 1959, 2:534.
73 Sinclair H. M., *The Work of Sir Robert McCarrison,* Faber, London 1951.
74 ——*Nutrition and Health,* Faber, London 1953.
75 Smith H. Williams, *J. Path. Bact.* 1965, 89:95.
76 Sokoloff B., Eddy W. H., Redd J. B., *J. Clin. Invest.* 1951, 30:395.
77 Stewart C. P., Learmonth J. R., Pollock G. A., *The Lancet* 1941, 1:818.
78 Tacquet A., Tison F., Devulder B., *Ann. Inst. Pasteur* 1961, 100:581.
79 Toomey E. G., White P. D., *Amer. Ht. Jour.* 1964, 68:841.
80 Turner E., Vickery K. O. A., *Vitalstoff-Zivilisations Krankheiten* 1966. 3:53.
81 Ungar G., *The Lancet* 1943, 1:421.
82 Walker A. R. P., Arvidsson U. B., *J. Clin. Invest.* 1954, 33:1358.
83 ——*Circulation* 1964, 29:1.
84 West R. O., Hayes O. B., *Amer. J. Clin. Nutr.* 1968, 21:853.

Appendix
The McCarrison Diet

A. A GOOD DIET AND A BAD ONE: AN EXPERIMENTAL CONTRAST

The investigation by Sir Robert McCarrison reported in the *British Medical Journal, Volume* 2, page 730, 1926, and the *Indian Journal of Medical Research,* Volume 14, page 649, 1927.

Two colonies of half-grown rats were employed, each comprising 20 animals of which 12 were males and 8 were females.

Details of the experiment:

One colony received 'a good diet', designed to resemble that eaten by the Sikhs. It consisted of chapattis, made of wholewheat flour; uncooked, green vegetables; fresh fruit (tomatoes, etc.); sprouted gram (legumes); butter; fresh whole milk; and fresh meat occasionally. A liberal allowance of butter was given spread over the chapattis; milk was supplied in amounts of approximately 300 cc daily; fresh meat was given every week to the amount of 2 oz for the whole colony. Liberal quantities of chapattis, sprouted gram, uncooked vegetables and tomato—to take the place of fruit — were given, so that the animals could select for themselves the amounts of each they cared to eat. Any food not eaten during the day was discarded when the cages were cleaned each morning.

The second colony received a diet which was ultimately shown to have been 'a bad one'. It was designed to resemble that eaten by many Western people of the poorer classes. It consisted of white bread, made from American white flour and obtained from the local bakery; vegetables—cabbage, carrot, potato, etc., cooked in water to which pinches of bicarbonate of soda and common salt were added; a substitute for margarine, consisting of coconut oil; tinned meat; tinned jam; tea, well sweetened with sugar, to which was added enough milk to give it the customary tinge; and water. The animals acquired an extraordinary liking for the tea; consuming as much as 600cc daily, and therewith approximately 20g of sugar and 20 cc of milk. Coconut oil was lightly smeared on slices of the white bread and the whole covered with a liberal coating of jam. The potted meat was given in like amount to the fresh meat in the first colony (2 oz weekly). Of the other ingredients of the food—the tea, the bread and jam and the cooked vegetables the animals were allowed to eat and drink as much as they liked.

The experiment was continued for six months. During its course the animals were kept scrupulously clean, and were comfortably bedded in fresh straw.

Results of the experiment: mortality

The mortality from all causes in the former colony was 15 per cent; in the latter 45 per cent. But whereas the survivors in the first colony were well grown, sleek-coated, strong and active, those in the second colony were ill-grown, poor-coated, weakly and listless.

Of the nine animals which died in the ill-fed colony, three were killed and eaten .by cannibalism.

The immediate cause of death in the other six animals was broncho-pneumonia; and this at a time when broncho-pneumonia was so rare in McCarrison's stock animals that only three cases of the disease occurred during the six months in a rat population which averaged at that time 375 daily. One consequence, therefore, of the 'bad diet' was to lower the resistance of the lungs to attacks by microbic agents of disease: a consequence of faulty food, deficient in vitamins.

Other post-mortem findings

Of these the most constant and the most important were changes in the gastro-intestinal tract which impaired its functional capacity, with extreme dilation and thinning of the whole gastro-intestinal tract; atony of the bowels; ballooning and transparency and intestinal stasis.

Fertility

Twenty litters were born in the well-fed colony during the six months the experiment lasted. In these 20 litters there were 134 young, all of which were reared to maturity. In the ill-fed colony two litters were born during the first few weeks of the experiment. One litter consisted of seven, the other of four. Of the eleven young, none survived.

Conclusions

This experiment demonstrated that a diet composed of whole wheat, milk, milk products, sprouted legumes, uncooked vegetables and fruit, with fresh meat occasionally, far surpassed in nutritive value that composed of white bread, tea, sugar, margarine, jam, boiled vegetables and tinned meat. Not only·does the former promote physical efficiency and health but the latter gives rise to stunting of growth, to physical inefficiency, and oftentimes to disease. The maladies of which the bad diet is so apt to lay the foundations are lung disease and gastro-intestinal disease. The high incidence of lung disease in the ill-fed group emphasized no less strikingly the influence of what one may call the 'white bread, margarine and tea diet' in favouring the operation of pathogenic agents which attack the lungs.

262

Author's note:

The good diet fed to McCarrison's rats led to a truly remarkable health record among his laboratory stock. Maintaining 1,190 stock rats on a diet consisting of a wholewheat flour, unleavened bread (chapattis) lightly smeared with fresh butter, sprouted Bengal gram (legume), fresh raw carrots and cabbage, unboiled whole milk, a small ration of raw meat with bones once a week, an abundance of water, both for drinking and for washing purposes, McCarrison observed no case of illness amongst these rats, no deaths from natural causes and no infant mortality.

Performing the post-mortem examination on these rats he encountered no macroscopical evidence of disease. The rats were kept in roomy netted-wire cages, screened and straw-filled in which they lived comfortably. housed.

McCarrison commented that it may be that some of them had cryptic disease of one kind or another, but if so, he failed to find either clinical or macroscopical evidence of it. He goes on to state, 'disease and death have been excluded almost completely by minute attention to three environmental conditions: cleanliness, comfort and food.'

B. THE DIET ITSELF

Sir Robert McCarrison emphasized the five principal components of a good healthy diet to be as follows:

(1) Whole grain cereals (e.g. wholemeal bread and muesli)
(2) Milk and milk products (cheese and yoghurt)
(3) Fresh vegetables
(4) Fruit
(5) Meat on occasions.

A recommended diet following these principles:

Breakfast:	Whole grain cereals (e.g. wholemeal bread and muesli), fruit and yoghurt.
Lunch:	A large varied salad with egg or cheese. Baked potato. Fresh fruit and yoghurt.
Supper:	A cooked vegetable dish, egg or cheese, or pulses (beans, peas, lentils), or whole grain brown rice. Fruit. Yoghurt.

Foods to be avoided include: all refined carbohydrates including white bread, biscuits, cake and sugar. Fried foods should be avoided also and fat consumption (cream, butter and eggs) well controlled. Meat, if eaten, should be light meat and lean.

Meat is not a daily essential if the diet is balanced. Sir Robert McCarrison recommended meat consumption about once a week, and recommended stock soups and lean meat.

It may come as a surprise to some that a complete amino-acid mixture is provided by a combination of raw greens in salad plus nuts. Sprouted grains and seeds are also good sources of vitamins minerals and proteins.

Where possible all processed foods and foodstuffs derived from packets should be replaced by the natural article eaten with the minimum of cooking or in the case of vegetables and fruit, as often as is feasible, raw.

C. THE McCARRISON SOCIETY

The McCarrison Society was formed in 1966 and originated from a need felt among doctors and dentists to form a society to study the aspects of nutrition put forward in this book, namely aspects of what is termed 'wholefood nutrition'.

Membership of the Society is open to doctors, dentists and nutritionists and those working in allied sciences. The aim of the Society is to provide a focus for activity in these fields, whereby study can be carried out into relationships between nutrition and health, the lessons from which can be applied clinically. Emphasis is laid upon the clinical approach, many of the current members being general practitioners and dentists.

The further aims of the Society are : —

(1) To emphasize the close link between sound nutrition and health, through regular meetings, conferences, and liaison with other societies.

(2) To encourage and initiate research projects in the field of nutrition and health.

(3) To collect and publicize available evidence relating to all aspects of nutrition and health.

The Society would welcome enquiries concerning membership. The address of the present secretary is :

Dr. B. Latto, 5 Caversham Road, Reading, Berks.

Index

269

John G. Eccles, Henderson Road, Longman Industrial Estate, Inverness.